TEACHING DURING ROUNDS

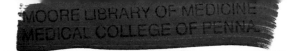
TEACHING DURING ROUNDS

A Handbook for Attending Physicians and Residents

DONN WEINHOLTZ, Ph.D.
College of Education, Nursing, and the Health Professions
University of Hartford
&
JANINE C. EDWARDS, Ph.D.
Department of Surgery
St. Louis University School of Medicine

Consulting Medical Editor
LAURA M. MUMFORD, M.D.
Department of Medicine
The Johns Hopkins University School of Medicine

THE JOHNS HOPKINS UNIVERSITY PRESS
Baltimore and London

For the attending physicians and residents
whose teaching we studied

© 1992 The Johns Hopkins University Press
All rights reserved
Printed in the United States of America on acid-free paper

The Johns Hopkins University Press
701 West 40th Street
Baltimore, Maryland 21211-2190
The Johns Hopkins Press Ltd., London

Library of Congress Cataloging-in-Publication Data

Weinholtz, Donn, 1949–
    Teaching during rounds : a handbook for attending physicians
and residents / Donn Weinholtz and Janine C. Edwards ; consulting medical editor, Laura M. Mumford.
        p.   cm.
    Includes bibliographical references and index.
    ISBN 0-8018-4351-0 (pbk. : alk. paper)
    1. Medicine—Study and teaching—Handbooks, manuals, etc.
I. Edwards, Janine C.   II. Mumford, Laura M.   III. Title.
    [DNLM: 1. Clinical Medicine—education—handbooks. 2. Teach-
ing—methods—handbooks. WB 39 W423t]
R834.W45 1992
610'.71'55—dc20
DNLM/DLC
for Library of Congress   91-35340

CONTENTS

FOREWORD

For centuries, a cornerstone of clinical education has been for medical students and junior physicians to make rounds on hospitalized patients with more experienced and professionally senior individuals. The form and substance of rounds have evolved over this time, and conducting rounds is now one of the most challenging academic tasks for contemporary physicians. It remains a task cherished by most, and it can bring an excitement to one's professional life. Challenge and excitement—these are the compelling forces confronting anyone who undertakes teaching during rounds.

The excitement of clinical education derives from the passion for medicine. Physicians, by providing medical care, enter a unique realm of interrelationships among themselves, patients, and illness. Navigating the resulting and sometimes turbulent diagnostic and therapeutic intricacies and providing high technology to interpersonal interventions that lead to safe harbor for some patients or tranquil sailing for others are exhilarating aspects of physicians' daily lives. When we allow ourselves to feel this exhilaration, when we embody it, how can we not have a passion, an excitement, for teaching our novice colleagues? Caring for patients includes caring for the learning of those who will care for patients after us.

Many of the challenges of teaching during rounds are well known. Dealing with students and house officers of varying abilities, varying levels of mastery, and varying degrees of motivation is a powerful challenge for all teachers—and an impediment for some. Being confronted with new clinical problems without the opportunity to prepare oneself for the teaching that derives from them can be threatening as well as challenging.

Creating learning excitement for another "routine" patient illness with which the team has had multiple previous experiences can be daunting. Integrating oneself with the tightly bonded house staff for a momentary time, reconciling who, in effect, is in charge, and establishing credibility with students and house officers are further challenges.

The greatest challenges, however, derive from two other potent dynamics. One is the newest requirement for rounds: the need for the attending physicians to do the business of patient care as mandated by legislation. Thus, attending physicians must use rounds to gather data about the patients under their care while simultaneously catching "teachable" moments to execute their responsibilities to educate. Residents who teach feel this same seemingly disparate pull between providing patient care and providing instruction at the same time. The second equally great challenge confronting any teacher on rounds is that of becoming integrated into a system of intense learning that develops from the novice professional's experience of providing patient care. The experience itself is a stimulating and demanding teacher, causing novices basically to educate themselves. The teaching physician typically steps into this rich learning environment after the fact, after the most powerful learning has occurred. Finding the aspect that further enriches the learning requires ultimate teaching skill.

It is small wonder that physicians feel tensions when they conduct rounds. Perhaps, to some extent, each eventually develops a strategy of teaching that provides the least personal tension. The strategy may be to overpower students and house staff with expert knowledge, or to rely on implicit modeling of professional behavior, or to entertain with stimulating behavior, or to devote one's energy to just providing patient care because of its priority over teaching. One marvels at those teachers who master the tensions and also teach effectively. During the past decade, the academic community has increased its awareness of these tensions and has put forth efforts to address them. It has created faculty development programs and has produced texts, conferences, and workshops on clinical education. All of these attempt to meet the growing demand of teaching physicians how to teach effectively. Even proposals for revising medical school curricula typically include programs to enhance the teaching effectiveness of the faculty.

This volume by Weinholtz and Edwards is a valuable addition to the resources available to teaching physicians. It is a handbook of alternative instructional strategies. These are strategies that attempt to convey the passion for medicine while reconciling the tensions derived from the challenges of teaching during rounds. It is indeed a "how-to" manual, based on accepted principles and conclusions derived from educational research. It provides a starting point for anyone interested in the improvement of personal teaching skills during rounds. Adhering to the suggestions does not guarantee success as a teacher. It guarantees a method of self-assessment, of experimentation, of increased versatility. It articulates the tensions, and it suggests ways to overcome them. The application of the suggestions will vary with the skills and sensibilities with which the teaching physician is already endowed. This handbook begins this enrichment process.

The passion for medicine and the desire to teach are inexorably linked. Both demand excellence. Caring for patients and caring for each other's learning while being steadfast in one's devotion to the alleviation of human suffering from illness are the professional ethos to which we are compelled to aspire.

LAURA M. MUMFORD, M.D.
The Johns Hopkins University School of Medicine

PREFACE AND
ACKNOWLEDGMENTS

For each of us, this book is the culmination of more than a decade's research, reflection, and writing about clinical teaching. During that time, one of us focused primarily on attending physicians' instructional efforts and the other focused mainly on teaching by residents. However, the instructions provided by attending physicians and by residents are so intertwined that neither of us could neglect the other's domain. Thus, it made good sense to combine our efforts in a book that addresses teaching by both parties.

We have tried to provide a thorough examination of the existing literature in the hope of accomplishing two goals: (1) to develop a practical handbook that attending physicians and residents can turn to when looking for guidance in developing their teaching and (2) to spur other educational researchers to examine a most intriguing and important area of investigation. By no means does our current awareness of what constitutes effective teaching during rounds fully and accurately represent the complete range of possibilities. Undoubtedly, there are new discoveries to be made, areas of confusion to be clarified, and mistaken assumptions to be refuted. Much good work remains to be done, and we urge others to get involved.

Throughout the book we have tried to provide clear illustrations of the teaching practices that we are advocating, as well as some that we oppose. These are all real-life examples taken either from our own observational and interview research or from that of others. To minimize redundant citations, we have presented many examples without providing references. Unless otherwise noted, illustrations dealing with teaching by attending physicians were taken from Weinholtz (1981), while those dealing with teaching by residents were taken from predominantly unpublished materials collected by Edwards at Louisiana State University and at St. Louis University. To assure the anonymity of the individuals included in these examples, pseudonyms replace actual names throughout.

Although some other texts have admirably addressed clinical teaching (Schwenk and Whitman, 1987; Douglas et al., 1988), we believe this book to be unique in its depth of coverage of a particular type of teaching, that occurring during rounds on hospital inpatient services. We greatly admire those who have already finely honed their teaching skills in this setting and those who are systematically attempting to do so. An extensive analysis of the arena in which they work seems warranted. We hope that, upon reading our effort, those to whom this book is targeted will agree.

We benefited immeasurably from others as we conducted our research and wrote this book. D.W.'s interest in attending rounds was sparked and nurtured by the troika of Frank Stritter, Bill Mattern, and Chuck Friedman. Then, over the years, Harold Levine, Mark Albanese, and Leo Harvill provided invaluable support for ongoing work. J.E. feels similar appreciation for Robert Marier, Frank Svec, and Warren Plauché, who shared their insights about teaching and learning, and for Damon Climes and Daniel Yips, two residents who provided both comaraderie and many good examples.

Early segments of our manuscript were typed by Donna Sabin and Gwen McIntosh at the University of Iowa. Later, Ginny McKinney at East Tennessee State University faithfully typed several versions of the complete book.

On the editorial side, Anders Richter of The Johns Hopkins University Press brought us together and launched this project. When Andy "graduated" to his retirement, Wendy Harris ably guided us to completion. Throughout, Laura Mumford's medical editing provided a reality check and valuable suggestions for two Ph.D.s writing about physicians.

Finally, our families deserve many thanks for all that they do for us.

TEACHING DURING ROUNDS

CHAPTER ONE

The Medical Team: A Teaching and Learning Group

Various formats and settings for clinical teaching are found in the modern teaching hospital. Grand rounds, lecture halls, outpatient clinics, and other settings are all worthy of study for the sake of improving one's clinical teaching. This book is designed to help readers better understand and improve teaching in one particular setting: the inpatient ward. The primary emphasis is on attending rounds, the daily teaching/working sessions conducted by attending physicians, but attention is also given to work rounds, the daily review of patients overseen by the service resident.[1] Conference room, hallway, and bedside teaching are all addressed. Also, teaching outside of rounds is addressed to the extent that it affects rounds. Throughout, the focus is on rounds as they traditionally occur on inpatient services in departments of internal medicine and pediatrics. This chapter describes the conditions that make teaching during rounds both distinctive and demanding. The remaining chapters offer specific suggestions for addressing these demands.

Effective clinical teaching requires that the instructors provide optimal patient care while enhancing the learning of the trainees assigned to them. Despite the inherent educational value of clinical settings, combining these two functions is no easy task. For example, few instructional formats are as ver-

1. A medical service may sometimes be assigned two residents who share management responsibilities. For example, one resident may take primary responsibility for teaching while the other is primarily concerned with overseeing patients. At a few teaching hospitals, two attending physicians split attending responsibilities along similar lines. However, the norm remains a single attending physician and a single resident. This is the configuration that we assume throughout the book.

satile and productive as attending rounds, which provide a vehicle for planning daily hospital work, training graduate and undergraduate medical students, and informing attending physicians on medical content outside their subspecialty areas. Combining the seclusion of the conference room with the rich interaction of a hospital ward, attending rounds allow for small-group instruction on immediate and compelling problems. They also foster valuable sharing and confrontation among members of the medical team. For all of these reasons, attending rounds are an extraordinary instructional invention.

The very things that make attending rounds an exceptional opportunity for education render them a demanding challenge for teaching. The months spent staffing inpatient services may be a faculty member's most taxing times of the year. The attending physician not only oversees the care of many very sick patients but also faces the problem of teaching various levels of learners, each with a dramatically different educational need. This teaching occurs in the face of a fluctuating patient census and periodic shifts in medical team personnel. Surely, few teaching assignments are as complex. No wonder wide variations in the quality of teaching on attending rounds have consistently been reported (Reichsman et al., 1964; Daggett, 1977; Mattern et al., 1983).

To address this complex type of teaching, we culled recommendations from the growing body of research on clinical teaching that has appeared since the early 1960s. No comprehensive theory of clinical teaching drove our selection of these recommendations, as no such theory yet exists. Consequently, we focused on the many research findings consistent with well-established learning principles. We also viewed teaching during rounds as an exercise in team leadership involving periodic shifts between teacher-centered and learner-centered instructional approaches and an overall progression from directiveness to delegation by attending physicians and residents (Weinholtz, 1981; Weinholtz and Friedman, 1985). Teacher-centered approaches involve a great deal of either teacher talk or teacher control of group discussion. The teacher is very directive. Learner-centered approaches allow learners much greater freedom in developing the instructional agenda. The teacher delegates substantial responsibility, and learners teach themselves and each other. Readers wishing more insight into this particular leadership perspective will find the underlying theory described in some detail in Chapter 8.

To illustrate briefly the value of a leadership perspective, we can examine one issue clearly demanding leadership during rounds: the use of time. Attending physicians and residents must regularly decide whose needs will be met and how time will be spent. The constant and compelling demands of patient care may cause important instructional procedures to be shunted aside and lost along the way (Weinholtz, 1981). The attending physician and resident must exert leadership using the authority stemming from their positions and their knowledge to ensure that sufficient instruction occurs throughout their team's time together. Patients' needs must never be slighted, but creative uses of time must be sought to make learning more than just some mysterious osmotic process. This book illustrates how certain attending physicians and residents recognized as outstanding teachers have ensured sufficient time for teaching and learning. We believe that other attending physicians and residents can improve their own teaching by studying these practices and adapting them for their own use.

Other factors affecting team members' educational experiences are the relationship between the attending physician and the service resident and the interplay of the remaining team members. Teams that function well tend to take on a corporate identity, with members forming loyalties to their leader and to each other. Members within such teams accept and execute their responsibilities, and they help one another. The educational merits of this sort of cooperation are apparent. Consequently, among the recommendations in this book are many leadership practices for promoting optimal team development.

Of course, individual personalities always influence the medical team's dynamics, but much of what happens is dictated by the interplay of formal roles (Miller, 1968; Mumford, 1970; Weinholtz, 1981). The remainder of this chapter presents sketches of the different team members derived from the medical education literature addressing the roles of medical students, interns, residents, attending physicians, and other health professionals. These sketches form a backdrop against which the recommendations offered in the remainder of the book can be understood more clearly. Medical students, interns, residents, and attending physicians are presented first, as they are the mainstays of rounds and the greatest amount has been researched and written about them. Other health professionals are discussed afterward because they participate in rounds less frequently and comparatively little study on their roles within rounds has been done.

Medical Students

Third-year medical students are the initiates on the medical team. As novice clinicians, they occupy the lowest rung of the service's authority ladder, but it is a position they do not hold for long. Within two years they become interns, and a year later, residents.

While the medical student's role is less influential than that of the other members of the medical team, it is not unimportant. During their clinical clerkships, students are socialized to hospital norms and begin developing the history-taking, diagnostic, treatment, and management skills that they will rely upon throughout their professional lives. Furthermore, the data collected by medical students on the patients assigned to them are used for diagnostic and management decisions. These data must be collected promptly and must be accurate. Students may develop both good and bad habits while carrying out these early responsibilities.

Although there are now many more women and minority students in medical school, a remarkable number of variables have remained constant in clinical clerkships since Becker, Geer, Hughes, and Strauss (1961) published *Boys in White,* their classic, participant-observation study. Becker et al. emphasized that "students absorb medical culture in a selective fashion as it helps meet the problems posed by their school environment. Thus what they use of medical culture is by no means the same as, or simply a junior version of the culture of the practicing physician. Rather it contains characteristic distortions and omissions which . . . account for many disagreements, both overt and implicit, between students and faculty" (p. 192).

As one would expect of adult learners (Knowles, 1973), medical students pursue what they perceive to be in their personal and professional self-interest as they are confronted with the demands imposed on them during the clinical clerkship. The bulk of these demands deal with aspects of "working up" patients. This involves taking the medical history, performing the physical examination, and making the differential diagnosis based on the history and the related diagnostic evidence (e.g., lab results, x-ray films, etc.). Typically, an intern oversees each student's patient-related work. Most of the students time is spent on the service, but supplemental seminars, lectures, and conferences are usually required.

Becker et al. (1961) identified the primary problems confronting medical students as sorting out what to study and learn, dealing with faculty, and dealing with fellow students. Becker et al. found that students seek knowledge and experiences that they view as immediately applicable to the practice of medicine. Accordingly, students tend to value the "pearls" of information provided by house staff and attending physicians. They also judge clinical services according to the range of patient conditions provided. Finally, they seek the responsibilities of making decisions and performing procedures in the face of some immediate danger to the patient.

Medical students tend to direct their efforts toward increasing both their clinical experiences and their medical responsibility. When frustrated in their attempts to do so, they encounter substantial tension and strain. Since clinical clerkships frequently involve the repetition of basic tasks over and over again, student tension and strain tend to mount over time (Becker et al., 1961).

Students tend to be sensitive to faculty demands and to modify their behavior to satisfy the faculty. Becker et al. found that students view faculty as examiners, disciplinarians, and controllers of academic fate. They observed that student subservience to faculty wishes is most clearly apparent during attending rounds, where students appeared willing to put up with anything and suffered from recurring fears of making a bad impression. Students often viewed faculty as capricious and demanding, but student resistance involved little more than bickering and gossiping behind faculty members' backs. Thus, they contributed to and expanded the reputations that preceded attending physicians on all teaching wards.

Finally, Becker et al. reported a fairly high degree of student cooperation. Viewing themselves as experiencing a shared struggle, students showed a remarkable willingness to help each other during both the basic science and the clinical years.

Subsequent research has tended to elaborate upon the description offered by Becker et al. without dramatically altering the original view of medical students' inpatient clinical experiences. Still, a few findings deserve mention. Coombs (1978) reported that students viewed clinical faculty with greater respect than basic science faculty and that students viewed house staff as preoccupied with their own learning experiences. However, students were tolerant of house staff because they identified with the house staff's heavy workload, and students were appreciative of whatever instruction house staff provided. The only house staff scorned were those who overloaded students with meaningless chores ("scutwork"). Even though students often viewed their clerkships as "helter-skelter" experiences and they seriously disliked "scutwork" and the "follow-the-leader" nature of attending rounds, they valued clinical education far more than basic science education. Also, students greatly enjoyed clerkships that were carefully organized to ensure a wide range of learning experiences. In spite of students' preferences to the contrary, Foley, Smilansky, and Yonke (1979) observed students repeatedly placed in passive roles "in which they received a preponderance of low-level, factual information." Although Weinholtz (1981) reported student experiences and levels of satisfaction varying substantially with the attending physician's teaching approaches, the Association of American Medical Colleges Report on the General Professional Education of the Physician (GPEP) (1984) noted the tendency of clerkships often to evolve into "unguided apprenticeships" in which students "inappropriately invest their time in routine patient care at the expense of their general professional education."

If there is ever widespread adoption of innovations in medical education like the alterations in clerkship structure implemented in the New Pathway at Harvard (Harvard Medical School, 1989), medical students' roles in clinical clerkships may begin to change, but evaluative data on the restructuring of clinical clerkships have not yet been reported, and "more than 98% of the medical schools in the world" remain "established and traditional" (Kaufman, 1989). For the time being, medical students' roles and experiences during most in-service clerkships seem unlikely to change. Variations in students' educational experiences will be affected primarily by the instructional approaches adopted by attending physicians and residents.

Interns

Interns occupy an important transitional role within the medical team. Although not far removed from medical students, they nonetheless are physicians, charged for the first time with major responsibility for patient care. While instruction during attending rounds may often focus on medical students' needs, work rounds predominantly address the problems and issues confronting interns.

In a 1961 time study, Payson et al. found that more of the observed interns' time was spent in staff communication than in any other activity. Given interns' needs for consultation and supervision, the researchers were not surprised by this finding, yet they did not anticipate the small amount of time that the interns spent with patients. The investigators reported that "the doctors spent barely enough time with their patients to establish an acquaintance, much less a relation." Furthermore, "there was a very rapid decrease in the amount of time spent with a patient after the first day of admission." Payson et al. speculated that interns diverted attention from patients to colleagues because of the interns' needs to obtain security and approval, acquire specific medical technique and knowledge, learn how to relate to other professionals, and focus on the diagnostic and pathophysiologic aspects of medicine.

Again, findings and interpretations offered nearly three decades ago are remarkably accurate today, and intervening research has tended to elaborate upon rather than to alter the basic picture. One participant-observation study found that, even though interns were not spending great amounts of time with patients, they were indeed involved heavily in patient care, typically at the expense of their academic activities (Miller, 1968). When interns found that they could not do everything that fell within their responsibility, they decided that academic responsibilities were the most readily expendable. As their experience increased, the interns were increasingly likely to miss attending rounds when conflicts with patients' needs occurred. Also, they progressively cut back on the reading necessary for turning rounds into lively intellectual sessions. Finally, through their questioning strategies interns attempted to "manage" their attending physicians, to keep rounds focused on immediately practical issues. It is apparent that the interns' reluctance to follow an attending physician's instructional lead may constitute a distinct barrier to learning on a medical service.

In another participant-observation study focusing on internships at both a university hospital and a community-based hospital, Mumford (1970) reported a distinct difference in interns' attitudes toward attending physicians according to the type of hospital. At the community hospital, where attending physicians controlled access to patients, interns accepted the attendings as role models and rarely challenged their authority. On the other hand, at the university hospital, interns looked more to residents as role models because the residents were more likely to be informed on the latest medical advances across a wide range of areas and the setting provided substantial opportunities for informal interactions with the residents. The cohesion between interns and residents at the university hospital was somewhat intimidating for attending physicians, especially those not employed full-time in the academic setting. Interns tended to view these "private practice" physicians as coming to learn rather than to teach.

As did the other researchers previously mentioned, Mumford noted a lack of emphasis among interns on establishing doctor-patient rapport. She also indicated no lack of concern for patients, but rather an overwhelming dedication to the notion that patients could best be helped if their physicians studied and discussed the facts surrounding the patients' diseases. Weinholtz (1981) argued that this preoccupation of interns with biomedical facts plays a substantial role in determining medical teams' norms during attending rounds, as residents and attending physicians often allocate time to respond to interns' perceived concerns rather than to alternative issues and problems such as the psychosocial aspects of medicine. The issue here is one of degree. In tertiary care centers, biomedical topics may easily predominate, even when psychosocial concerns are the cause of the patient's illness or dysfunctional state.

This focus on biomedical knowledge to the exclusion of physician-patient relationships is compounded by the intern's work overload. The Association of American Medical Colleges' (1981) report, *Graduate Medical Education: Proposals for the Eighties,* emphasized that interns "are often expected to carry case loads and hours of duty that stress their mental and physical capacities" and that such demands may be contrary to good education, training, and patient care. Furthermore, interns not only are responsible for expanded case loads, but also have taken on additional, burdening responsibilities likely to tax even the most capable individuals. For example, Mangione (1986) argued that she had been well prepared by medical school for much of what she was required to do during her first year as a resident in general internal medicine but that she was quite unprepared for her responsibilities: "(a) teaching medical students; (b) functioning as an effective ambulatory care doctor; (c) dealing with the psychosocial issues surrounding terminal illness, death and dying; and (d) functioning as a cost-conscious member of the medical system."

Clearly, medical students and interns provide an attending physician or a resident with two distinct groups of learners whose special needs must be addressed. Residents too, however, have unique learning needs and provide a third level of instruction that attending physicians must deal with when they teach. We will now explore the residents' role on the medical team.

Residents

Miller (1968) found that the reliable source of power for residents when supervising interns' patient care was the great inequality of information between the two groups. Typically, residents simply knew much more about medicine and about the hospital than did the interns. Residents thus advised new interns, and the interns were placed in their debt. However, Miller noted that by the sixth month of the internship there was a shift in the relationship, with interns resenting too much infringement on their responsibilities. The resentment was checked somewhat because interns realized that they too would soon be residents, and they did not wish to undermine the status of the positions they would soon hold. Residents typically responded by trying to maintain friendly, egalitarian relationships with interns to obtain smooth operation of the medical service through the use of personal influence rather than by resorting to their tentative authority.

Focusing on the relationships between residents and attending physicians, Daggett (1977) found that, although the resident and attending physician were supposedly a team responsible for patient care and teaching, in practice each suffered from little understanding of the other's role. "Furthermore, the lack of definition of roles of these two key people on the ward tended to produce either a competition between the two for the position of ward manager and/or withdrawal by one or the other to a position of relative non-involvement" (Daggett, 1977, p. 106).

In Daggett's study, all members of the medical team viewed the resident as the service manager, which required being knowledgeable about all patients, acting as a liaison between hospital staff members, being up to date on research, and coordinating opportunities for the teaching of trainees by the attending physician. Attending physicians in the study viewed effective ward residents as great aids, but ineffective residents as individuals "to be monitored constantly, and sometimes overruled in decisions."

Finally, Daggett reported that the relationship between the attending physician and the resident was often so blurred that the attending physician was not viewed as a supervisor who was truly responsible for the medical service and on occasion was not even viewed as a member of the service team. Indeed, interns and medical students rated their interactions with residents as more important learning experiences than their interactions with attending physicians. These findings were consistent with those from a participant-observation study conducted by Bucher and Stelling (1977), who reported that, as their experience increases, residents increasingly place greater weight on their own judgments regarding the quality of their performances than on the judgments of their attending physicians.

Unlike the literature on medical students and interns, the literature focusing on residents moves beyond attitudes and relationships to examine residents' teaching. The importance of such teaching has been greatly emphasized in recent years. The Association of American Medical Colleges (1981) urged that residency programs be designed in a manner to enhance residents' abilities to teach and to evaluate their students. Also, various approaches to developing residents' teaching skills have been reported by medical educators throughout the last decade (Lawson and Harvill, 1980; Jewett et al., 1982; Camp et al., 1985; Edwards et al., 1986, 1988b; Edwards and Marier, 1988).

Apter et al. (1988) found that most residents enjoy teaching and consider it a critical component of their own education because teaching increases their medical knowledge. Many (42%)

of the respondents to this survey indicated that attending rounds were their least satisfying teaching setting, an understandable finding, since residents generally play second fiddle to attending physicians during attending rounds. However, two studies yielded data somewhat unfavorable to residents teaching during work rounds, the setting in which residents exhibit the greatest control over instruction (Wilkerson et al., 1986; Wray et al., 1986). In the first, Wilkerson and colleagues observed that residents relied on a restricted range of teaching behaviors, rarely referring to the literature, giving feedback, demonstrating techniques and procedures, or asking questions. In the second study, Wray's team reported that data-collection efforts and reviews of vital sign sheets and medication sheets during work rounds were insufficient for ensuring proper patient care, much less for providing a sound basis for instruction.

Even when a resident's data-collection efforts and teaching skills are maximized, the issue of how teaching duties will be shared between the resident and the attending physician remains. The distribution of these teaching responsibilities greatly influences the quality of students' and interns' instruction, as well as the resident's overall satisfaction with the teaching experience (Weinholtz, 1981). The manner in which the attending physician approaches his or her role critically influences the amount and direction of the residents' teaching.

While both attendings and residents are important role models for medical students and interns, attendings in particular can teach students, interns, and residents how to relate well to patients and families, refine history-taking and physical exam techniques, solve medical problems, and manage patients. Explaining the pathophysiology of medical conditions and stimulating curiosity to learn about a disease process in depth are additional important teaching tasks of attendings. Also, teaching complex skills, such as surgical procedures or interpretation of specialized imaging studies, is usually reserved for attendings because of their greater experience and expertise.

Residents, on the other hand, can complement attendings' teaching in a variety of ways. Because residents are with students and interns so many hours every day, they can demonstrate and supervise the practice of basic clinical skills. Students must plod through detailed histories and physical exams with many patients to routinize the information to be gathered and the sequence of the gathering. They must see basic procedures performed, and they must have guidance while practicing these procedures themselves. Residents can elicit basic science knowledge from trainees and assist them to relate it to clinical signs and symptoms. They can also assist students in the process of formulating differential diagnoses. Drug dosages and lab values are probably best taught by residents, who are in constant contact with these detailed facts. Finally, work habits, such as thoroughness, accuracy, and punctuality, can be taught by residents, who are on the scene constantly.

Attending Physicians

The medical education literature focusing on attending physicians has primarily addressed the quality of attendings' teaching efforts. Unlike the attitudes of medical students and interns, attendings' attitudes toward their role and responsibilities have received little attention, and the literature on attending physician teaching has ignored the difficult balancing act that a university faculty member performs during a month spent attending. Typically, although not true at all teaching hospitals, the attending physician must oversee patient care and thus is legally responsible for the management of all patients on his or her service. In addition, the attending is charged with teaching the several medical students and interns assigned to the service as well as with instructing the service's residents. The attending also probably sees clinic patients once a week, perhaps gives a few guest lectures throughout the month, supervises or participates in data collection on one or more research projects, attends several committee meetings, works on one or two journal articles or book chapters, tends to various administrative chores, and attempts to maintain some sort of personal life. Needless to say, the months spent attending may be the most stressful times of a faculty member's year.

Clinical settings provide tremendous opportunities for instruction but also place unique demands upon attending physicians. Indeed, the literature on teaching during attending rounds often appears quite paradoxical, yielding many findings indicating the virtues of such teaching but also revealing many shortcomings. Comparing basic science classroom instruction with clinical instruction, Jason (1962) found that clinical instructors were better able to "challenge" their students by focusing on case discussions and stimulating interest via their own questioning, prodding, provoking, and reflecting comments by students. Indeed, the small-group, attending-round setting is ideal for this sort of teaching, and Coppernoll and Davies (1974) reported that attending rounds are a learning format highly valued by medical students. However, while observing 82 clinical teaching sessions, 56 of which were attending rounds, Reichsman et al. (1964) unearthed many problems with teaching during attending rounds. Even though attending physicians saw patients with students in three-quarters of the attending rounds, they often missed opportunities "to make significant observations or to show meaningful interaction" between the attending and the patient. In the overwhelming majority of observed rounds, students were not asked to conduct any part of the physical examination or to interview the patient even briefly. In half of the cases, attending physicians did not even briefly interview patients to evaluate data previously presented to them by students. On the other hand, a few attendings allotted an extreme amount of time for "painstaking, detailed" patient examinations, thus leaving little time for other teaching objectives.

Reichsman et al. also noted a striking lack of basic science teaching, apparently due to attending physicians' difficulty staying current in basic science knowledge. In one half of the rounds, clinical syndromes and concepts were clearly taught; in the remainder, however, either the discussion of such topics lacked clarity or they were not taught at all. Furthermore, in one third of the rounds, case presentations did not form the basis for discussion of differential diagnosis, and more than one-quarter of all sessions generated insufficient and irrelevant medical information. Finally, in only one-fourth of the observed sessions did clinical teachers stimulate students to acquire knowledge by suggesting or assigning textbook material or other medical literature.

Reichsman et al. attributed many of the observed shortcomings to the shear enormity of the teaching challenges confronting clinical instructors. They stated: "We believe that the difficulty of this task is unique in the entire realm of teaching. In no other field does the nature of the teaching material demand of the teacher this degree of preparedness without preparation. We suggest that the problem of learning how to teach as a clinician deserves much thoughtful study if the clinical teacher is to survive as a highly competent and respected scientist."

A host of observational studies conducted during the 1960s, 1970s, and 1980s provided support for the findings of Reichsman et al., indicating that some problems with attending physicians' teaching have remained fairly constant (Adams et al., 1964; Payson and Barchas, 1965; Hinz, 1966; Daggett, 1977; Tremonti and Biddle, 1982; Mattern et al., 1983; Maxwell et al., 1983). However, research has also shed light on what makes certain attending physicians excellent teachers. For example, surveys by Stritter et al. (1975) and Irby (1978) provided general dimensions that learners associated with effective clinical teachers. Stritter et al. reported that such teachers provide a personal environment in which students are active participants; maintain a positive attitude toward teaching and students; concentrate on the problem-solving process; use student-centered instructional strategies; demonstrate a humanistic approach showing sensitivity to individual patient needs and encouraging students to share feelings, values, and experiences; and emphasize references and research. Irby found that effective clinical teachers are organized and clear, capable group facilitators, enthusiastic and stimulating, knowledgeable, clinically competent, capable supervisors, and professional role models.

Some specific criteria for helping attending physicians improve their teaching emerged from more recent research attempting to develop quantitative assessments of the effectiveness of attending physicians' teaching by examining correlations between particular instructional approaches and specific measures of effectiveness (Petzel et al., 1982; Skeff et al., 1985; Weinholtz et al., 1986a). The applicability of these criteria were examined in other studies evaluating efforts to improve attending physicians' teaching (Skeff, 1983; Medio et al., 1984; Skeff et al., 1984; Tiberius et al., 1987; Weinholtz et al., 1989).

Drawing on the growing literature examining attending physicians' and residents' teaching, this book offers recommendations for addressing the instructional challenges provided by rounds. There is mounting evidence that teaching during rounds can be modified and that such modifications are appreciated by both students and teachers (Skeff, 1983; Edwards et al., 1986; Tiberius et al., 1987; Edwards et al., 1988a, 1988b; Weinholtz et al., 1989). Such change can occur if attendings and residents are willing to reflect on their teaching, are open to suggestion, and are committed to experimenting with different teaching behaviors.

Other Health Professionals

In a survey of 123 directors of internal medicine residency programs, Weinholtz et al. (1986b) reported that 49 percent of the 111 responding directors indicated that only attending physicians, residents, interns, and medical students regularly participated in attending rounds within their departments. On the other hand, 34 percent indicated that clinical pharmacists were regular participants, 18 percent reported the same of nurses, 8 percent acknowledged physician assistants, 4.5 percent included medical social workers, and 5.5 percent claimed regular involvement by other sorts of health professionals.

Often nonphysicians are relegated to relatively passive roles during medical rounds. The neglect of these individuals is well illustrated by the fact that there are virtually no references to nonphysician health professionals in the entire body of literature addressing either attending rounds or work rounds. However, there is an increasing awareness of the value of teamwork involving physicians working more closely with other health professionals. The GPEP Report of the Association of American Medical Colleges (1984) specifically called for multidisciplinary teaching rounds and team-building experiences to enhance students' teamwork skills.

Daily rounds may provide a rich interdisciplinary teaching laboratory where teamwork skills can be developed. While providing a challenge to the status quo and yet another consideration placed upon attending physicians and residents, the instructional possibilities of interdisciplinary rounds are particularly exciting.

Summary

If one observes attending rounds or work rounds, one cannot escape noticing the different levels of authority and expertise present. The perspectives held by the participants and the underlying dynamics of the work group are not nearly as apparent. This chapter, by focusing on the literature addressing the different subgroups of the medical service team, has sketched a general picture of these more elusive factors.

Medical students are initially thrilled by their exposure to real clinical experiences, but they soon tire of repeating routine functions. Although continually seeking new experiences and responsibilities, they often feel overlooked by house staff and intimidated by attending physicians. Feeling as though they cannot take much initiative, many medical students slip into passive roles.

Although they possess a medical degree, interns are still advanced apprentices who are initially overwhelmed by the medical responsibilities confronting them. Anxious to obtain the medical knowledge necessary for dealing with their patients' immediate problems, they actively pursue what they perceive as useful information or skills and become frustrated when diverted from their course (e.g., when an attending physician allocates a great deal of attending round time to address students' needs). Also, the interns' focus on getting the "right medical answers" often causes them to lose sight of important psychosocial, patient-management issues.

Residents occupy a position between the students and interns on one hand and the attending physician on the other. They are viewed by all as the service managers, who are expected to conduct work rounds and facilitate attending rounds in cooperation with their attending physician. Typically, the manner in which residents are supposed to perform their responsibilities is not clearly defined, and residents must "wing it," adjusting to the skills of the individuals below them and the whims and capabilities of the attending physician. Both the resident and the attending physician are likely to experience confusion and frustration if their relationship does not evolve according to their expectations.

Attending physicians are assigned the difficult task of providing leadership in patient care while teaching all levels of learners within the team. This role is intimidating and often forces attendings into offering the detailed medical information desired by interns. Frequently, attendings can provide only the level of detail they perceive as desirable within their own subspecialties. Thus, they tend to focus on subspecialty knowledge rather than to emphasize broader knowledge or the general clinical skills that are time consuming to teach.

Other health professionals frequently are present during attending rounds, but their participation has too often been minimized while the agendas of physician team members are pursued. We believe this situation tends to perpetuate the isolation of physicians from their fellow health professionals and stifles opportunities to use rounds for team-building purposes.

These are the underlying dynamics with which attending physicians and residents must deal when teaching during rounds. The remainder of this book draws on the research conducted over the last three decades to offer specific suggestions for dealing with these dynamics and for attempting to optimize the educational benefits for all involved.

CHAPTER TWO

Starting the Rotation

At 9:30 A.M., Dr. Jeffries met in the conference room with the three medical students assigned to his service. It was Dr. Jeffries' first day as the team's attending physician, but the students had already been on the service for five days. Displaying a friendly, collegial manner, Dr. Jeffries asked the students to identify the interns with whom they had been working. He also asked them the names and diagnoses of their patients, the content covered during attending rounds by the previous attending physician, and any content areas they needed to learn better. As the students responded to his questions, Dr. Jeffries carefully listened and jotted notes on their comments.

After collecting this information, Jeffries explained that he would be "splitting" rounds to enable him to teach the students and the house staff most effectively. This would involve meeting alone with the students at 9:30 A.M. before the rest of the team joined them at 10:30. He would also meet with the students from 2:30–3:30 on Tuesday and Wednesday afternoons. The morning sessions would be reserved for presentations of the previous day's patients and for visiting patients' bedsides. The afternoon meetings would deal with in-depth discussion of some of the more common problems on the floor. These sessions would also be used for the students to make presentations to each other on various topics. Jeffries gave the students a list of topics from which to choose and informed them of resources available to them to research their chosen topics. The topic list included coronary artery disease, chronic obstructive pulmonary disease (COPD), alcoholic liver disease, diabetes, peptic ulcer disease, hypertension, leukemia, and lymphoma.

Concerning their patient presentations, Jeffries told the students to make them concise, focusing on the chief complaint followed by the pertinent positives and negatives. He carefully explained why conciseness and precision are important to case presentations. He also described a list of procedures that he and the house staff would be teaching during the month. Jeffries then closed his orientation session by asking the students if they had any questions of him, taking time to respond thoroughly to each student's concerns.

The Attending Physician's Responsibilities for Orientation

The session just described shows an attending physician taking the time to ensure that the medical students on his team clearly understand his expectations for them during the rotation. He also took the opportunity to gather information from the students to assess their learning needs. In doing so, he demonstrated the three key recommendations of this chapter.

1. Clearly orient all team members to your expectations for the rotation.
2. Negotiate agreements with team members to develop learning activities consistent with their abilities, interests, and expectations for the rotation.
3. Establish a climate conducive to learning.

The rationales for these recommendations follow, accompanied by illustrations and suggestions for implementation.

Stating Expectations

As indicated in the previous chapter, several studies reported confusion within medical teams because of uncertainty and misconceptions regarding the attending physician's expectations for rounds (Reichsman et al., 1964; Daggett, 1977; Weinholtz, 1981; Mattern et al., 1983; Medio et al., 1984). Often team members adopt a "wait-and-see" attitude, with the first few days of the rotation spent in a trial-and-error mode as the team adapts to the attending's style. Of course, a certain amount of apprehension and tentativeness is unavoidable whenever a group is forming under the guidance of a new leader. However, through more careful planning and communication, overt problems such as the one illustrated in the following case can be avoided.

Jim, the senior resident, had been asked by Dr. Livingston, the attending physician, to explain to the students how they should deliver their case presentations. Livingston made this request without previously conferring with Jim about how Livingston would like the presentations done.

Jim obliged. Meeting alone with the students after the first day's rounds, he told them to keep their presentations to seven minutes, rather than fifteen, and to save time by skipping the negatives on the physical exam.

The next day Dr. Livingston commented to Charlie, the medical student who was about to begin his presentation, "Remember to keep it to fifteen minutes, and don't leave out anything."

Obviously surprised by this message, Charlie asked, "Do you want to hear all of the negatives?"

"Yeah, I don't mind listening to them," answered Livingston.

Charlie proceeded, somewhat nervously attempting to fill in the negatives that he had not expected to have to present.

Mix-ups such as that just described can easily be avoided if the attending physician takes time to orient the team to key expectations right at the start, rather than as problems arise. In a national survey, Schor and Grayson (1984) found that most individuals recognized as outstanding clinical teachers do so. Medio et al. (1984) demonstrated that additional time spent by attending physicians on establishing ground rules, expectations, and the purposes of rounds is perceived as a clear improvement of teaching behavior. Weinholtz and Ostmoe (1987) suggested how a clinical teacher can facilitate such orientation sessions by providing (1) a brief overview of the role of the rotation in the students' and house staff's medical education, (2) the attending's view of the team members' clinical responsibilities, (3) assumptions about the entry level capabilities of the various levels of team members and learning objectives for each level, (4) an explanation of how the attending will evaluate team members' performance, (5) highlights of any particular hospital policies or regulations that the attending wants emphasized, and (6) any supplementary information that the attending wants to include, such as key journal references, text citations, or other information resources.

These points can simply be reviewed orally with the team at the start of a rotation. Some attendings may want to generate a document to ensure that team members have received key information in writing. Although considerable thought and effort must be invested when creating such a written guide, once the initial work is done only minor revisions are likely to be necessary to keep it up to date.

Given the team's varying levels of abilities and needs, it can be valuable for the attending physician to meet separately with the students, the interns, and the resident to spell out expectations and negotiate agreements regarding instruction with each set of learners. By doing so, the attending can ensure appropriate education for each level of trainee. Of course, the attending should also share expectations and negotiate agreements appropriate for the team with the entire group.

One final point regarding expectations deserves special emphasis: evaluating a learner's performance is one of the most sensitive and crucial tasks confronting a teacher. Motivation is affected markedly by the way learners feel they are going to be judged. As Ways and Engel (1982) documented, too often students in clinical settings feel that they are evaluated capriciously and arbitrarily. Interns and residents also report similar concerns (Weinholtz, 1981).

One way that attending physicians can base their evaluation efforts on a sound foundation is to give careful thought beforehand to the criteria that they will use when judging team members' performances for purposes of assigning grades or writing evaluations. But careful thought alone is not enough. The criteria should also be clearly articulated to the team members. For example, if "negatives" are to be included in presentations, that should be stipulated. If psychosocial issues are to be included in formulating the differential, that too should be clearly specified. If the attending is going to judge the residents' ability to organize and deliver a brief lecture, the criteria should be articulated. It is easy to ignore these sorts of considerations. Many teachers do. However, clear communication of such details is one of the things that makes an excellent teacher. What Erickson (1984) stated regarding classroom instruction also holds true for clinical teaching.

> The intimate connection between goals and grades is frequently overlooked. It is inconsistent, for example, to proclaim you are teaching students how to think, to solve problems, and to discriminate values but then to test achievement in terms of the ability to memorize. One acid test of the internal consistency between goals

and testing is the linkage between pronouncements made the first day of class and the kinds of questions on the final examination. Consistency is a matter of fair play, and students should know from the beginning what standards are to be met at the end of the course. (p. 16)

Soliciting Information from Team Members

In designing effective instruction, it is essential to gather information on learner characteristics before initiating planning efforts (Kemp, 1985; Dick and Carey, 1985). Proceeding to teach based solely on one's assumptions concerning learners' expertise, previous experience, and motivations is often an inadequate strategy because one's assumptions are often incorrect. Even with a fairly accurate notion of what to expect from most learners, teachers frequently encounter surprises from particular individuals. Asking team members for their own assessments of their abilities, their interests, and their expectations is an efficient way of collecting data for fruitful planning. For example, in the illustration at the beginning of this chapter, when Dr. Jeffries asked the students the topics covered by the previous attending and the content areas in which they felt somewhat deficient, he quickly identified some areas appropriate for brief lectures. Similarly, by asking the resident the role that he or she would like to play during rounds, an attending may avoid unintentionally frustrating the resident's expectations for sharing teaching responsibilities. If it turns out that the attending and the resident have different expectations, then at least both sets of expectations can be laid out for negotiation.

Establishing a Positive Climate for Learning

One reason for soliciting information from students is the straightforward collection of data for planning. A second reason is that information solicitation helps establish a climate conducive to learning by developing a norm of group participation right at the start of the rotation. Both students and house staff report that they value instruction that occurs in a comfortable environment in which they are active participants (Stritter et al., 1975). As the following comments illustrate, the tone set by the attending plays an important part in determining team members' reactions to their learning situations.

My experience on a service is pretty much determined by the attending. If rounds are an enjoyable learning situation, it can pick up your whole day, but if they are just another two hours of drudgery, then it just adds to the other 16 hours of drudgery that you have to go through. (Intern)

First of all, personality-wise, an attending has got to be confident. Second, I think that an attending has got to be friendly and outgoing because the stresses of the situation can be unbearable when you get a stone-face. Attendings have to have a sense of humor. (Resident)

Dr. Goff is very good. She's knowledgeable and personable, and she keeps rounds light. . . . No one feels that they are put upon. . . . They can speak without being attacked. . . . She encourages an open atmosphere where you can feel safe. (Resident)

Clearly, effective communication and supportive group leadership are important components of good clinical teaching. It is not our intent here to provide a primer on the skills necessary to maintain two-way communication and a supportive learning environment, but such skills are worth reviewing, developing, and refining. In particular, three skills described in detail by Gordon (1977)—active listening, I-messages, and no-lose negotiation—are worthy of close examination. Active listening requires that a listener restate in his or her own words the message expressed by the person to whom he or she is listening. By doing so, the listener confirms that the message was accurately heard and interpreted.

I-messages contain three components that combine to enable the instructor to convey efficiently and nonthreateningly his or her reactions to a learner's behavior. The components are (1) a brief description of the behavior found to be either acceptable or unacceptable, (2) a concise description of the instructor's feelings regarding the behavior, and (3) a precise explanation of the likely effect of the learner's behavior. (For example, "Brian, your consistent difficulty in getting along with patients and the nursing staff distresses me. Unless you show some improvement I will have to grade you 'unsatisfactory' in that area.")

No-lose negotiation is a conflict-resolution technique that fosters joint problem-solving efforts among participants. It requires using active listening and I-messages to ensure effective communication throughout the problem-solving effort. The six steps used in no-lose negotiation are (1) identifying and defining the problem, (2) generating alternative solutions, (3) evaluating the solutions, (4) choosing preferred solutions, (5) implementing the decision, and (6) following up to evaluate the solution. In the case illustrated above, the attending physician could implement no-lose negotiation to develop a plan whereby Brian could clearly demonstrate improvement in his relations with patients and the nursing staff. Other illustrations of communication skills used by teachers in clinical settings are provided by Douglas et al. (1988), Schwenk and Whitman (1987), and Weinholtz and Ostmoe (1987).

The Resident's Responsibilities for Orientation

The resident's responsibilities for orienting the students to the service and the learning experience are similar to those of the attending. The resident should

1. state expectations,
2. solicit information from students and interns for planning instruction, and
3. establish a positive learning climate.

However, much of what the resident does in these areas must take into consideration the approaches adopted by the attending physician.

Stating Expectations

Residents typically have greater control over many noninstructional, medical service matters. For example, they must establish work routines, such as regular times for work rounds, check-in and check-out rules, and the like. Most residents do this and consider it adequate communication about the expectations for students and interns. These work responsibilities are necessary, but not sufficient, in a learning environment; that is why we stress the need to communicate learning objectives.

In separate sessions with students and interns, the resident should reinforce the expectations stated by the attending physician. If the attending does not initiate such communication, the resident should make an opportunity to talk privately with the attending about these matters. The resident must find out the attending's expectations for both the resident and the other members of the team, including learning objectives and evaluative criteria.

The clerkship director may also communicate objectives and evaluative criteria for students to all residents and interns at the beginning of the academic term. If that communication is not initiated by the clerkship director, we recommend that residents take the initiative to find out the objectives and evaluative criteria of the clerkship. Then, of course, the resident should manage the patients and team so that the students have opportunities to attain their objectives. This may seem obvious, but the students' objectives can be overlooked on a busy service where residents must care for many patients, fulfill hospital regulations, and resolve conflicting time demands.

Perhaps the most important thing a resident must tell students is that they should ask for help when they need it. The only "sin" is not to ask for help. A patient's well-being, or even a life, depends upon this cardinal rule. Of course, the corollary to this is that the resident must be willing to give help when the students ask.

Soliciting Information from Students and Interns

Residents have a myriad of opportunities to solicit information from students about their medical interests, their aspirations, their fund of knowledge and procedural skill, their families, and their social lives. Because residents spend so many hours every day with the students on work rounds and working one on one with students, they can informally acquire a rich store of personal information. All of this information can be used to motivate students to learn, to delegate responsibility, and to target the resident's teaching, as in the following example.

After the attending left the ward team in the hall, Al, the second year resident said, "Well, noon conference has been canceled. Let's go get something to eat."

Sitting around a crowded table in the basement cafeteria, Al said to John, a third year student who was sitting across the table from him, "So you are from California? Do you find the Midwest very different?"

"Yeah, it's very different," said John, "but I haven't had time to do much that I could describe. The people here are more—conservative, monotonous. Their lives seem to be pretty dull. In California, we go surfing when we have a beautiful day! And we're only a couple hours away from the ski slopes. I used to go skiing all the time."

"Did you ever see any serious ski accidents?"

"Yeah, all the time. In fact, that's how I got interested in being a doctor. I want to be an orthopedist. I saw an orthopedist put a guy back together who I thought would never walk again."

Al made a mental note of this comment as the conversation turned quickly to someone else talking about his favorite ski trip.

Establishing a Positive Climate for Learning

Establishing a positive learning climate is an important, but elusive, task for the resident who heads the service. A collegial climate, where students and interns are regarded as junior colleagues, seems to promote learning among the team members. Each member of the team, of course, has responsibilities and must be accountable to the resident for those responsibilities. The climate should allow an open exchange of ideas and information between team members and the attending.

One way that a resident can promote a positive learning environment is to help minimize excessive gamesmanship during work rounds and attending rounds. Arluke (1980) described in careful detail the characteristics and functions of "roundsmanship." He found that the intellectual give and take during rounds is often used by team members to (1) manage impressions of their competence, (2) control the attending's instruction, (3) control the attending's supervision, (4) establish trust among peers, and (5) establish status among residents and interns.

There is a long tradition of roundsmanship within clinical medical education. As one of the residents in Arluke's study commented: "Roundsmanship sets the atmosphere. There is an atmosphere of competitiveness and one-upsmanship in a teaching hospital. . . . I don't care which one it is."

Within reasonable limits, such competitiveness can have beneficial instructional effects. However, if the one-upsmanship becomes excessive or if rounds too often stray into esoteric areas to allow particular individuals to display their arcane knowledge, then negative effects may outweigh benefits. Ideally, the resident should work with the attending to keep rounds focused on content relevant to the medical problems encountered on the service. Also, the demands made of team members should be evenly distributed so that each individual can shine or falter based on his or her own merits.

Combining Efforts for a Good Start

Orientation is a very important instructional requirement under any circumstances. In the complex world of the teaching hospital, where teaching responsibilities are shared and learners' tasks carry such important consequences, orientation becomes even more important. Attendings and residents must orient themselves to each other before they can successfully launch a team through an educationally sound rotation. This preliminary step can prevent unnecessary problems and create many exciting learning opportunities.

CHAPTER THREE

Allocating Time for Teaching

There are some attendings who don't . . . really work within the time schedule. They work at their own pace. I've had experiences with attendings who spend a lot of time on small talk, then the first patient is presented, then we go to the bedside to see the patient, then we go back and have a discussion. We spend almost forty-five minutes on each patient. If we have four or five patients, we can spend until one o'clock on rounds!

The above quotation from an exasperated resident draws attention to an important demand confronting clinical teachers, the judicious use of time. Clinical education is exceptionally powerful because it is experiential education grounded in work settings, but work settings are often hectic places allowing little time for the reflection and exploration that in-depth learning of complicated phenomena and medical procedures requires. The inpatient service is clearly this sort of busy work environment, but tradition has wisely preserved opportunities for medical team members temporarily to escape some of the commotion so that explicit teaching and reflective learning can occur. This chapter explores some of the steps that attending physicians and residents can take to make the optimal instructional use of these opportunities.

The Attending Physician's Allocation of Time

Although attending rounds are set aside as a time for teaching, pressing work demands such as those caused by a high patient census can often intervene to prevent much explicit instruction from occurring (Weinholtz et al., 1985). Even when attending round time is dedicated to instruction, there is the additional problem of finding enough time to address the various needs of the team's different levels of learners. In the search for additional time with the team, some attendings may join work rounds for all or part of the rounds. Others may devise alternative strategies. The existing literature relating to these two problems, preserving time for teaching and equitably distributing that time among the team members, leads us to the following recommendations.

1. Personally review charts and visit patients before attending rounds to reserve a maximal amount of attending round time for teaching.
2. Conduct special teaching sessions for medical students.

Reviewing Charts and Visiting Patients before Rounds

Typically, attending rounds allow a review of the status of the "old" patients (i.e., those admitted before the previous round), as well as the presentation and discussion of the new patients. At the discretion of the attending physician, the team may address the old and new patients for differing lengths of time in varying locations such as a conference room, in the hallway, or at patients' bedsides. Here we address the time issue. Recommendations concerning teaching in different locations are dealt with in Chapters 4 and 5.

One recurring instructional problem during rounds involves the review of old patients spilling over into the time set aside for the presentation and discussion of new patients, a period when a great deal of teaching usually occurs. This is not really a difficulty if changes in patients' conditions merit extensive discussion and provide substantial grist for instruction, but it is particularly troublesome if the review of old patients deals predominantly with the routine information already discussed by the team during morning work rounds.

An in-depth study of six attending physicians' teaching during rounds revealed distinctly different approaches for conducting the review of old patients (Weinholtz, 1981; Mattern et al., 1983). One attending consistently used more than thirty minutes, sometimes as much as forty-five minutes, for this review. Every morning he ran down the entire list of eighteen to twenty-four patients, asking the team to provide him with an update on each patient's status. Little, if any, overt instruction occurred during this time. The exercise appeared solely designed to keep the attending apprised of patients' conditions.

Three other attendings observed in the study also ran down the entire patient list but did so quite briskly, pausing only when a pertinent matter for discussion or instruction arose. This approach, which usually took fifteen to twenty minutes, minimized discussion of information redundant with morning work rounds, yet provided the team with opportunities to discuss and learn from important patient developments.

Finally, two other attending physicians, Dr. Waitzman and Dr. O'Leary, demonstrated a distinctly different strategy. These attendings, without relying on a list, asked the team questions pertaining to a few specific patients about whom they were concerned. They then asked their teams if there were any new developments about which the attendings should know. This approach reduced to an absolute minimum the exchange of information redundant with morning work rounds. Barring the need to discuss a major problem occurring overnight, these attendings were often able to finish their reviews of old patients in ten minutes. They could do so because they closely monitored the current status of the services patients' before attending rounds, thus minimizing their reliance on rounds to provide them with information and preserving substantial blocks of time for teaching.

These two attendings in particular conducted careful reviews of charts and made regular visits to patients' bedsides outside attending rounds. Although these activities would seem to be a basic part of every attending's professional responsibilities, the study mentioned here clearly revealed differences in the thoroughness with which attendings engage in such activities and the extent to which they consciously apply their knowledge of patients' conditions to the educational structure and content of their attending rounds.

One caution regarding careful monitoring of medical service patients by attending physicians deserves mention. While keeping close tabs on their services, attendings should generally avoid conveying the impression that they have lost confidence in the house staff's ability to care for the patients (unless, of course, certain individuals do not merit such confidence). The morale problems that can be created by an attending who is perceived as maintaining too much control are illustrated by a resident's remarks. "One attending that I had was one of the best attendings I have encountered, with the exception of the fact that . . . he kept calling me in the middle of the day to ask me the very fine details on our patients. Knowing these aspects were the intern's responsibilities, . . . I felt like he didn't really trust me. . . . It made me feel uncomfortable, and it made the other residents covering the service feel uncomfortable also."

The previously mentioned patient-monitoring practices of Dr. Waitzman and Dr. O'Leary contrasted particularly with those of Dr. Sampson, the attending who conducted a prolonged review of old patients each day. Dr. Sampson ritualistically used the review as a large portion of the time that he was expected to fill during rounds. This behavior seemed tied to his discomfort in pursuing other topics. He confessed: "I think that often I am not terribly effective as an attending. I think that, particularly when I get outside of my area of special interest and competence, I don't have a lot to say. I have trouble orienting the discussion, with the students in particular, in such a way that it is a learning experience for them."

Although a renowned laboratory researcher, Dr. Sampson did not have the finely tuned clinical skills of his other colleagues participating in the study. Drs. Waitzman and O'Leary, on the other hand, were highly credible clinicians who drew on their substantial clinical experience and their moment-to-moment awareness of their patients' conditions to create learning conditions highly valued by their team members.

Conducting Special Sessions for Medical Students

Teaching three different levels of learners is one of the challenges of attending rounds. As one attending physician put it:

> The remarkable thing about rounds is talking to people with three completely different levels of expertise and interest. . . . Students are somewhat virginal, if you will. They really want to hear a discussion of disease. . . . They also want to hear a discussion of what the physical findings mean, and how the physical examination works, and how history works. So it is very broad for them.
>
> The interns are less interested in basic mechanisms than time. They are more interested in what the major differential is and, more importantly, what to do and how to do it fast. . . . So they are concerned about management.

The residents are more aloof. Although concerned about management, and their concern is about doing things as rapidly as possible, they are more concerned with the broad picture. It's almost back to the students again. . . . This is their last year, and they want to hear broad differentials and they want to hear how tests are interpreted. . . . So they're really three quite distinct groups. It is almost like coming full circle in a way.

Various approaches for addressing the needs of these three different levels of learners have been reported (Weinholtz, 1981). These approaches can be grouped according to the attending physician's use of special sessions devoted specifically to the third or fourth year medical students. One approach involves meeting with the students before the department's designated (or suggested) time for starting rounds. For example, if attending rounds typically begin at 10:00 A.M., the attending could meet with the students from 9:15 or 9:30 until 10:00. A second approach involves conducting rounds at the standard time with the entire team but scheduling sessions during the afternoons with the students. A third approach involves beginning rounds at the standard time but requiring only the students to be present for the first half hour or so and the house staff to join after that. This approach preserves time alone with the students but tends to shorten attending rounds for the house staff. A final approach involves conducting attending rounds with the entire team present and not holding any sessions specifically for students.

No experimental research has been conducted on the merits of these various approaches, and attending physicians' rationales for adopting these various schedules reveal conflicting opinions regarding what can and what should be accomplished during attending rounds. For example, a well-respected attending physician who allocated a great amount of time to special sessions with students while still conducting standard-length rounds with both the students and the house staff present, commented:

It would be tedious for the resident to have to sit there and to listen to my critique of the student's presentation. . . . Actually, I think that they were very grateful to have that extra half hour so they could do their chores. . . . It also gave me the opportunity to actually go with the students to see the patient before the house staff came.

On the other hand, another highly respected attending, who did not conduct special sessions with students, offered this view.

People conduct rounds in various ways, as you have discovered. Some have a session with the students first and then with the house staff. That has never appealed to me too much because, although the levels of their training and education are highly different, I don't really find it too difficult to incorporate all of them into the same discussion. The idea that I have is to get each person to contribute according to his abilities, to the level of training that he has had, so that each one can feel like he is making some contribution to the care of the patient.

However, in the study where these various approaches were reported, both students and house staff indicated that they preferred having the attending physician meet separately with the students. Their sentiments are reflected in the following two comments focusing on having the students meet with the attending before rounds. The first comment is from a resident, and the second is from a medical student.

I'm glad that he is bringing the students in at 9:15. Otherwise you end up tearing your hair out. It gives the attending some time to work with the students on presentations, and not everybody has to sit through them. . . . The interns just need the time on the floor because they have so many tiny details to square away.

I think it's good. The only problem is that you're rounding from 8:00 until 12:30, but by 9:00 lab results aren't in anyway. The good thing about it is that it gives you a chance to present the patient without the intern there. When the interns are there, they have to add their own bits of information, and it throws off the presentation. This way you get feedback just on what you do.

In spite of their general approval, some house staff in the study perceived some drawbacks to the attending's meeting with the students before the beginning of rounds. First, they expressed a concern that the students might misinform the attending. Second, they were concerned that the attending might provide some useful information that the rest of the team would miss.

Having the resident present during the student sessions is a way to alleviate the first problem but not the second. However, one attending physician observed during the study adopted a strategy that addressed both problems. This attending, Dr. Jeffries, met with students before the rounds to listen to their case presentations. Immediately following a presentation, he took the students to the bedside to perform his own partial physical and to obtain a brief history from the patient. Later, when the house staff arrived at the conference room, either he had an intern provide a capsule summary of the patient presented by the student or he provided one himself from a thorough set of notes that he had taken during the student presentation. By doing so, Jeffries was able to keep the entire team informed while seeing if there were any major discrepancies between the student's presentation and what the intern knew of the patient. By keeping his capsule summary brief, Jeffries was able to minimize the redundancy for the students, at the same time providing them with a model of a concise presentation. Then, during a short follow-up discussion with the house staff he could also reiterate any key teaching points regarding the patient that might be of interest to the interns or the resident.

Beyond the strategies that have been reported in the literature, other possibilities certainly exist. For example, learning needs of the differing levels of team members might all be met through a learner-centered approach that attempts to get everyone involved by having participants alternate between teaching and learning roles. The attending can facilitate team members' instruction of each other by correcting or amplifying as needed. Interactions can all be very collegial and supportive. For example, after presenting the case the student is asked to critique his or her own performance. Following that, the interns and residents offer their critiques of the presentation and provide suggestions for improving it. Explicit feedback can briefly be modeled by the attending and developed by the other team members to everyone's benefit.

Next, the intern might be asked what his or her biggest concern was on approaching the case under discussion. The resident would then be asked to expand on those concerns, given his or her greater expertise. For example, what were the things that the resident wanted to be sure to check about the case to ascertain that the intern was not going astray? The differential diagnosis could then be developed, starting again with the student. Additional questioning of the student and intern about how well the differential diagnosis explains the case can provide the instructor with insight about the analytic skills of both levels of learners. The resident could then be asked to provide what he or she sees as the soft spot in their differential diagnosis. By that point, numerous possibilities for the bedside interaction would be evident. The team could then decide how they would address the deficiencies or critical features uncovered by the discussion to that point. The history and physical exam features for the bedside teaching could be identified so that everyone would be prepared for what would happen at the bedside.

The literature offers some valuable models for conducting rounds. However, individual attending physicians and residents must rely on their own creativity and assessments of their own situations when deciding how to pursue their teaching. The challenge of efficiently using time to meet the needs of the different levels of learners is just one of many opportunities for creative, new responses.

The Resident's Allocation of Time

We offer two recommendations to assist residents in allocating time for teaching.

1. Use "teachable moments" whenever possible.
2. Plan ahead.

To allocate time for teaching, residents must perform a complex juggling act. The resident who is in charge of an inpatient service has many responsibilities. He or she must supervise the care of all patients on the service, setting priorities and making adjustments as complications develop. The resident must assess the abilities of each member of the team and assign duties accordingly. The attending physician must be kept apprised of each patient's condition. Additionally, the resident is expected to teach the students and other residents and also to take a role in their evaluation. To accomplish all of this, the resident must manage time and the work process efficiently.

This individual and team allocation of time must be viewed within the larger context of the current debate about the total number of resident working hours. In 1984 the Libby Zion case in New York touched off a series of investigations into resident work time and working conditions that continue to have profound repercussions in United States residency programs (Asch and Parker, 1988). The tradition of residents working more than 100 hours per week in the hospital and clinics is being challenged by at least two forces: (1) the desire of the public and the medical profession to improve the quality of patient care and (2) a growing demand by physicians for more time for leisure and family.

An editorial in the February issue of the *Journal of the American Medical Association* boldly proclaimed that there was no turning back from fundamental restructuring of residency training, which should include reduced working hours, improved ancillary services, hours better distributed, increased participation of attendings, uniform requirements with "teeth," restrictions on moonlighting, and anonymous reporting of violations (McCall 1989).

The Accreditation Council for Graduate Medical Education has mandated that residents work no more than eighty hours per week, have one day out of every seven days off, and be on call no more than every third night. Internal Medicine residency programs are struggling to implement these new regulations. A "night float" on-call system and nonteaching services are two mechanisms being tried. This experimentation is perceived by traditionalists to cause interruption in continuity of patient care and to decrease the amount of training with patients that residents receive.

However, Lurie and associates (1989) published a time study of resident and intern activities while on night call. They found that residents and interns spent only a small portion of time on direct patient care activities but much time on writing in charts and doing procedures and other tasks that could be performed by nonphysicians. This study presents evidence that questions the value of night call for patient care training. No attention was given in this study to documenting the amount of time residents and interns spent teaching each other or medical students.

Use Teachable Moments

Our observations of resident teaching activities indicate that valuable teaching can take place during unscheduled times (i.e., those times not scheduled for work rounds, attending rounds, morning report, and the like). When students are working alongside residents to admit new patients and to carry out the orders for patients assigned to the team, residents have many opportunities to teach spontaneously. Taking advantage of these "teachable moments" is the best recommendation we can make. The following example illustrates how such teaching can take place.

One afternoon Bob, an internal medicine intern, passed Jane, a third year medical student on his team, in the hall of one of the medicine services. Jane stopped him and said that the Digoxin level of one of her patients was at a low therapeutic level.

"Should I increase it or leave it alone?" she asked.

Bob asked, "Why is she on Digoxin?"

Jane replied, "To control her heart beat. She had atrial fibrillation."

Bob said, "Yes, but she doesn't have it anymore. Digoxin doesn't convert the rate from atrial fibrillation to a normal rate, but it controls the rate. She converted on her own."

Jane said, "Her heart beat is 65."

Bob said, beginning to edge away, "I would definitely not increase it, but discuss it with Estelle (the intern responsible for Jane's patient)."

Interns and residents can teach many things in the heat of action. Students have a need to know and are, therefore, highly motivated to learn. Residents can impart information and also teach communication patterns, as Bob did.

Plan Ahead

Our second recommendation is to plan ahead. Plan the activities for the succeeding day at the close of the current day. During the day, adjust the plans to meet changing exigencies. Some residents do this naturally. Others are so overwhelmed by the demands of the current day that they lose awareness of the value of explicating organization. We observed Dr. Whusthem, a senior pediatrics resident, organize her team regularly. She rounded up her team in the afternoon before the students left for their four o'clock lecture. She checked on the work each person had been assigned to do and previewed the next day's schedule with the team. This included scheduled activities for the students, such as lecture and attending rounds, and morning call and conference for the residents. She set the time and place for the team to meet the following morning. This gave everyone a sense of order. As the day unfolded, the plan was adjusted to fit exigencies.

Those residents who are members of a ward team need to plan their patient care activities and study time around the team activities. Thinking ahead about when during the next day, for example, to perform a lumbar puncture and when to grab an hour of reading time can make these activities happen. The resident can then arrange with the student to assist and learn the procedure. Of course, something may intervene at those planned times, and then the resident must adjust the plan. Without such plans, time for teaching and reading frequently disappears.

Making the Most of What Is Available

Effective clinical teaching demands efficient management of time. There is so much to be accomplished on inpatient services within teaching hospitals that time can easily slip by without much instruction occurring. The learning needs of all team members must be addressed. To maximize learning, attending physicians and residents must wisely plan the uses of their time and take advantage of teaching opportunities as they arise. At first glance this task may appear overwhelming, but many outstanding clinical teachers manage to rise to the task. Through conscious effort the time can be found and the instruction can occur.

CHAPTER FOUR

Teaching in the Conference Room

The conference room, the hallway, and the bedside are the three locations where most teaching during rounds occurs. Attending physicians in particular are likely to allocate one half or more of their attending round time to conference room sessions (Schor and Grayson, 1984). Residents are more likely to conduct work rounds in the hallway and at the bedside (Wilkerson et al., 1986), but they too may reserve some time for the conference room. In this chapter, we explore a variety of ways that both attendings and residents can enhance the quality of their teaching in the conference room. In the next chapter, we focus on teaching at the bedside and also address teaching in hallways.

The Attending Physician's Teaching in the Conference Room

We have five recommendations for attending physicians.

1. Limit interruptions of the case presentations by students and house staff, reserving the majority of questions and comments until after the presentations are completed.

2. After case presentations, actively engage in discussions, using probing questions to assess understanding and to provoke thought.

3. Frequently use illustrative devices (e.g., chalkboard, x-ray viewer, EKG tape, etc.) to emphasize important information and make abstract points more concrete.

4. Deliver occasional, brief talks on pertinent topics from the attending's subspecialty area or on general topics in which the attending is particularly well versed.

5. Provide team members with relevant readings or references and encourage team members to share information obtained through their readings and consultations.

Limiting Interruptions during Presentations

What I have found over the last several years is that many of the students don't like to be interrupted when they are presenting a case. . . . Sometimes they have the story as sort of a single piece within their mind. They start in, and they want to get through the whole thing. Then, when they are done, they are ready to talk about it. If you interrupt in the middle of that piece, it throws them off. I've seen students get completely thrown off so they couldn't organize their thinking or present a problem clearly at all. . . .

But if you don't interrupt them, a small piece of information or a minor issue that you will not return to may not be addressed. So, I will often tell them that it is my habit to interrupt people. But I won't do it if it is clearly upsetting their train of thinking. . . . The other reason that I like to be able to interrupt is because early on, if they present me with a piece of historical information and I can't tell why they are presenting it or it isn't clear to me what they are presenting, then I can get clarification. . . .

If they don't want you to interrupt, then you have to wait until the whole story is over and mentally make notes of the points that you want to come back to with the student. What I find is that I can't remember all of the points and I don't get back to them. So some opportunities are missed for interaction with the student. So the question is, "Can you interact with the student while the student is telling you the story?"

This attending's comments illustrate some of the difficulties inherent in listening to case presentations while trying to teach the presenter. These problems are most apparent when students are the presenters. However, a parallel though less dramatic situation occurs when interns present.

Many of the interruptions initiated by attending physicians come in the form of questions. It may be helpful for attendings to distinguish between "clarifying" and "probing" questions (Weinholtz, 1983a). A clarifying question may be defined as one the instructor asks to ensure her own understanding of what the presenter has communicated, as in the following examples.

"Exactly how much weight did you say that she lost?"

"Is that the scar from the prostate operation?"

"Could you summarize his medicine again for me?"

"How did she describe the pain?"

"Do we have the most recent x-ray?"

A "probing" question may be defined as one the instructor asks to determine the extent of the learner's knowledge or understanding or to provoke thought. Such questions may be asked to assess the learner's ability to grasp factual knowledge, comprehend key concepts, apply basic principles, analyze complex situations, or evaluate courses of action.

"What does hepatomegaly indicate to you?"

"Is that systolic gap significant, and what can you do about it?"

"What does the word 'diffuse' mean in histologic terms?"

"Do you think that the first doctor who saw her should have performed a pelvic exam?"

"What is the normal creatinine level in a patient this age?"

Attending physicians' styles of questioning during case presentations can be categorized according to the frequency of the questions and according to the relative use of clarifying and probing types of questions. Frequency can be categorized as low, medium, or high, and the types of question can be categorized as clarifying, probing, or mixed. A matrix showing all combinations of these two variables yields nine possibilities (Table 1). The four cells marked in the matrix indicate the questioning styles used by the attending physicians observed at a ma-

Table 1. Instructors' Questioning Styles during Student Presentations

Type of Question	Frequency of Question		
	Low	Medium	High
Probing			•
Mixed	•	•	
Clarifying	•		

Source: Weinholtz, D. (1983) Directing medical student clinical case presentations. *Medical Education*, 17:364–368.

jor medical center (Weinholtz, 1983a). The other five styles were not observed in the study, nor has any subsequent research reported on their effectiveness.

Table 2 provides a description of the advantages and disadvantages of the four observed styles of questioning. The high-frequency probing style contained some clarifying questions but was dominated by probing questions that tended to fluster and disorient the students during their presentations. Students reported having trouble thinking while confronted with a "barrage" of questions. For example, during rounds one student was frustrated when confronted by his instructor with many questions that he could not answer. He turned to the resident and blurted: "Well, respond, or do something! Give me some clues. Can't you see that I am struggling?"

This instructor's students, however, also reported that his questioning drove them to their books to do further reading. As one student indicated: "Nothing shames and embarrasses me like being asked a question that I can't answer. . . . That has happened to me more on this service than on any other. It's kind of like pledging a fraternity. You hate it the whole time but, even though you hate it, you feel like you are getting something out of it. When I am asked a question, I'll go and look it up, and read on it, and I learn."

The medium-frequency mixed style of questioning contained a better balance of probing and clarifying questions, seemed less disruptive of students' thought processes, and was apparently stimulating. As one student indicated after a presentation marked by such questions: "Even though he'll interrupt you while you are presenting, he doesn't throw off your thinking. Some instructors just ask you so many questions that you can't think, and you end up not learning anything."

Another reported: "I like him because he is no nonsense. He asks questions, but they are pertinent questions. He makes you work hard, but you learn a lot."

When instructors used low-frequency mixed styles of questioning, students generally expressed appreciation and stated their preference that most questions be held until after the presentation. Nevertheless, a few interruptions were viewed as only a minor obstacle. As one student indicated: "My normal inclination is to want to do my presentation without being interrupted at all. I've done presentations for people who interrupted me and got me totally confused, but this instructor only asks a few questions, and he can do it without disturbing me."

Finally, there is the low-frequency clarifying style of questioning. This style was illustrated by an instructor who, while asking a few questions, kept busy taking a thorough set of notes on each patient presented. The instructor reported that he consciously did not interrupt. "I avoid interrupting in order to give them the opportunity to present themselves. If you are taking a history from a patient, the best way to gather the information is to have the patient tell you his own story, rather than giving him leading questions and sidetracking him. The same is true when you are trying to assess a student. Quite frankly, there were times when I had to literally bite my tongue to not interrupt."

Because of his notes, this attending physician was able to ask comprehensive questions of the students when they had completed their presentations. As they were not trying to present information and answer questions at the same time, students generally responded to the questions without signs of confusion. One student reported that the instructor's note-taking behavior made the student realize the importance of the presentation. The student felt that the note taking reinforced the need for accurate communication, as it was apparent that the instructor was "actually comprehending" what the student was saying.

Based on the research conducted to date, it appears that either a low-frequency/clarifying or a low-frequency/mixed style of questioning is generally preferable when receiving presentations from students, and it is quite likely that these are also the best approaches when listening to presentations by house staff. However, more frequent use of questions may be desirable when encountering the occasional problem student who consistently comes to rounds unprepared.

Using Probing Questions during Follow-up Discussions

The discussions following case presentations provide rich opportunities for assessing the depth of team members' knowledge as well as for provoking them to think about particular problems and issues. Probing questions seem particularly well suited for these tasks. In one study, frequent use of such ques-

Table 2. The Advantages and Disadvantages of Different Styles of Questioning

Style of Questioning	Advantages	Disadvantages
High-frequency probing	Provokes student into carefully preparing presentations	Flusters and disorients student, thereby inhibiting instructor's ability to assess depth of knowledge and presenting skill
		Prolongs presentations and rounds
Medium-frequency mixed	Enables instructor to assess depth of student's knowledge and ability to present a case	Most difficult approach to implement, as optimal number of probing questions is hard to gauge
	Provokes student to prepare carefully, while stimulating interest	

Low-frequency mixed	Enables instructor to assess very selectively depth of student's knowledge, while providing very clear indication of ability to present a case Easy approach to implement	If left unguided, student may ramble, consume time, and bore other team members
Low-frequency clarifying	Provides clearest indicator of student's ability to present a case Most preferred by students	If left unguided, student may ramble, consume time, and bore other team members Instructor must take notes or concentrate very carefully to remember follow-up questions

Source: Weinholtz, D. (1983) Directing medical student clinical case presentations. *Medical Education*, 17:364–368.

tions by attending physicians was significantly correlated with overall ratings of teaching effectiveness completed by both medical students and residents (Weinholtz et al., 1986a). However, the attending again must beware of stringing together too many probing questions, thereby confusing or even panicking team members. A single question is often sufficient to evoke situations highly conducive for teaching.

> Following one student's case presentation, Dr. Livingston turned to a second student (Abe) and asked, "So, based on what you have heard, what type of obstructive disease does Mr. Ketchum have?"
>
> Abe quickly generated a list of possibilities including asthma, COPD, emphysema, and chronic bronchitis, but he displayed the limits of his knowledge when he had difficulty eliminating any of the possibilities. Abe grasped at emphysema but somewhat exasperatedly acknowledged that it was only a guess.
>
> Recognizing that additional questions might only further fluster Abe, Dr. Livingston acknowledged that emphysema was the correct diagnosis and demonstrated how the other possibilities could be ruled out. Then Livingston pointed out how Mr. Ketchum had been on a steroid inhaler, which could be quite detrimental to him considering his emphysema. He stressed a key point to the entire team.
>
> "Remember, you always ought to think 'Does he have a disease?' before you treat him. Otherwise you end up treating symptoms. Don't end up treating symptoms or you'll get burned every time. The patient may end up much worse off from all of the medicines he is taking. Simply treating symptoms is shotgun medicine and you ought to avoid it."

One straightforward probing question launched this entire sequence of events with instructional value not only for Abe but also for the rest of the team. Previous experience had taught Dr. Livingston that Abe was easily flustered by repeated questioning. Thus, he chose not to place excessive pressure on Abe when he was already demonstrating some confusion. Additional questions may have been appropriate with another student or with Abe at another time. A different brief encounter illustrates this point.

> After Susan completed her presentation of a patient with substantial respiratory problems, Dr. Goff asked, "Looking over the list, what do you think she might have?"
>
> "Sarcoid?" responded Susan questioningly.

"Sarcoid! What does sarcoid have going for it?" Goff quickly asked.

"Well, it's a restrictive type of disease," came Susan's reply.

"What percent of sarcoids don't exhibit a problem x-ray?" followed Goff.

Susan sat there stumped, so Al, the resident, chimed in, "Thirty percent."

"Therefore a chest x-ray is important because seventy percent of sarcoids have a problem," Goff said emphatically.

In this case, the attending delivered three questions in quick succession, again pressing the student to the limits of her knowledge. Once reaching that point, the attending used the situation to make an important clinical point. This sort of adroit use of probing questions is an important skill in clinical teaching.

Using Illustrative Devices

Because extensive information is exchanged during rounds, it is important for attending physicians to direct learners' attention to particular points worthy of special notice (Stritter and Flair, 1980). This, of course, can and should be accomplished through verbal emphasis, but other useful ways of highlighting important information involve using the various illustrative devices at hand such as the chalkboard, the x-ray viewer, or the records generated by diagnostic tests such as electrocardiograms or echocardiographs. These devices also serve to make abstract points more concrete. Such "illustrating" seems to be an important instructional behavior that correlates with ratings of teaching effectiveness completed by team members at all levels (Weinholtz et al., 1986a).

The chalkboard is usually the most versatile illustrative device available. It can be used to sketch diagrams of particular conditions such as lesions, nodules, or an enlarged rather than a normal heart. It also is quite useful for listing problems, possible diagnoses, diagnostic tests, or treatments. Skeff et al. (personal communication, 22 December 1991) found that teaching behaviors that bring about self-directed learning, by evoking learner's own personal thoughts, interests, and goals, that is, brainstorming, were correlated with positive learner outcomes. Quick brainstorming exercises can be used to develop comprehensive lists of diagnostic problems and management procedures from which appropriate clinical decisions can be made. Team members, particularly house staff, have reported the value of such an approach. As one resident indicated: "I like the attending to orient the discussion toward the patient's problems by outlining the problems. I like him to list them on the board and then to discuss them one at a time, giving the intern, resident, or student a chance to give the differential on each of the problems." Another reported: "When I was an intern, I had an attending who was really excellent. She would go through the whole case and, as we were going through the list of important problems, she would put them down on the board. Then she would put a flow sheet on the other side in which she would show the things that would lead from the problems. That was really helpful."

Table 3 shows a chalkboard illustration for a single patient recorded by an attending physician during rounds. After listing the organ systems himself, the attending asked questions whose answers allowed his team to fill out the remainder of the chart. During this process, the team members (three students and a resident) carefully pondered possible entries and actively contributed their suggestions.

Another approach for using the chalkboard was suggested by Russell (1985), who developed a technique called "condition diagraming" which is especially well suited to the systematic organization of case discussions. When listed on the conference room chalkboard, a condition diagram provides team members with a thorough but concise overview of the patient's past, present, and potential status. Figure 1 is Russell's schematic presentation showing the components of a condition diagram.

Figure 2 is a simple illustration used by Russell to show what a condition diagram might look like for a real case. An attending could record a diagram such as this on the chalkboard while asking the team to generate the diagram's four lists.

Because of time demands, attending physicians might typically use the chalkboard in a more limited fashion than either of the ways just illustrated. This sequence of events is a case in point.

> Dr. Waitzman: "Before we go to see her, for the benefit of the students, let's put down on the blackboard the things that she might have."
>
> (Dr. Waitzman draws out the following information from the team and records it on the board.)

Table 3. The Chalkboard Listing Used to Facilitate Problem-solving Efforts during Rounds

Organ System	Symptom	Disorder	What to Do
Cardiac	Wide aorta/diastolic insufficiency	Aortic insufficiency	Echo/phono
Genitourinary	Hesitancy/dribbling	Benign prostatic hypertrophy	Acid phosphatase/urology consult
Neurologic	None	Thrombosis	Review old scan
Gastrointestinal	Dysphagia	Esophageal motility disorder	Manometrics
Respiratory	dyspnea on exertion/orthopnea/wheeze	COPD/emphysema/monilial pharyngitis	Pulmonary function tests/stop steroid inhaler

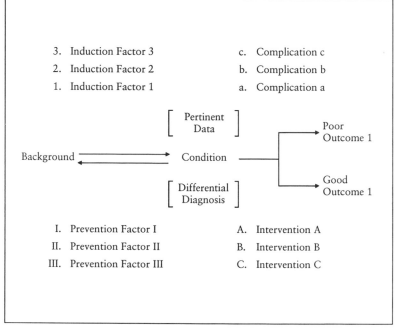

Figure 1. Schematic of a Condition Diagram
Source: Russell, I. J. (1985) Condition diagramming: A new approach to teaching clinical integration. *Medical Education,* 19:220–225.

Pulmonary Hypertension
1. Pulmonary parenchymal disease—Sarcoid
2. Occlusive disease of pulmonary arteries
    a. Pulmonary emboli
    b. Pulmonary arterial lesions
        —Pulmonary hypertension
        —Lupus
        —Scleroderma
3. Left-side heart disease
    —Mitral stenosis
4. Left-to-right shunt

In a follow-up interview, Dr. Waitzman indicated that he used the chalkboard in this manner to ensure obtaining a quick, but systematic, overview of disease possibilities. Although done primarily for the students' benefit, the exercise also was a helpful review for the house staff.

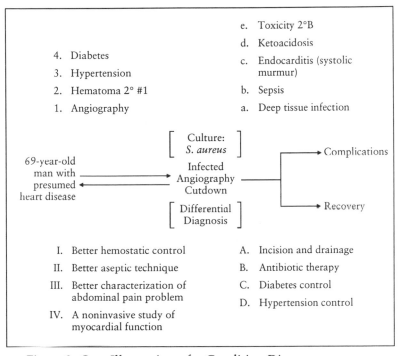

4. Diabetes
3. Hypertension
2. Hematoma 2° #1
1. Angiography

e. Toxicity 2°B
d. Ketoacidosis
c. Endocarditis (systolic murmur)
b. Sepsis
a. Deep tissue infection

69-year-old man with presumed heart disease → Infected Angiography Cutdown [Culture: S. aureus] [Differential Diagnosis] → Complications / Recovery

I. Better hemostatic control
II. Better aseptic technique
III. Better characterization of abdominal pain problem
IV. A noninvasive study of myocardial function

A. Incision and drainage
B. Antibiotic therapy
C. Diabetes control
D. Hypertension control

Figure 2. Case Illustration of a Condition Diagram
Source: Russell, I. J. (1985) Condition diagramming: A new approach to teaching clinical integration. *Medical Education,* 19:220–225.

Delivering Occasional Brief Talks on Pertinent Topics

The retreat from the bedside to the conference room as the primary setting for attending rounds is a cause for concern frequently expressed in the medical education literature (Engel, 1971; Linfors and Neelon, 1980; Brownell and McDougall, 1984; Shankel and Mazzaferri, 1986). Indeed, it is vitally important that the team not remain overly confined to the conference room. Attending rounds should not become a set of presentations, discussions, and lectures far removed from the patients on the service. However, the educational benefits that can be derived from judicious use of the conference room must also be acknowledged and exploited for their full value. As the following comments from two interns show, didactic presentations can have an important place during rounds.

I think that the most useful thing that an attending can do is to present minilectures when a new patient is presented or when a new twist occurs with one of the old patients. It is really helpful when they share their knowledge.

Giving talks is one of the areas where the attending can help us most. There really isn't enough time to read, so it helps to be able to get information like that. It is much more helpful than simply running through the patients.

Several studies reported team members' preferences for brief, focused didactic presentations delivered by attendings (Mattern et al., 1983; Maxwell et al., 1983; Schor and Grayson, 1984; Weinholtz et al., 1986a). These studies indicated that the attending physician should not let such presentations dominate rounds. Rather, the talks should be brief, spread throughout the month, and focused on topics pertinent to the patient problems encountered on the service. Topics from either the attending's subspecialty area or general medicine are likely to be appropriate as long as the talks do not stray far from what the team views as immediately relevant. One way the attending can keep his or her talks on target is to alert team members at the beginning of the month to several topics on which the attending is prepared to present. The team can then choose the topics they would like to have covered, and the attending can deliver the talks at opportune times in conjunction with discussions of appropriate patients. This approach was used by Dr. Livingston and was particularly appreciated by the house staff, as indicated by one of his two residents' comments: "Among Dr. Livingston's strengths is the fact that he has taken the time, on occasion, to prepare special talks. . . . He took the time to run over pulmonary function tests for the whole group, and he also did the same thing on pulmonary diseases and the complications of certain drugs."

Of course, it is also possible for the attending to give brief, spontaneous talks as appropriate moments arise. However, again the attending should exercise caution and not allow this practice to get out of hand and occur too often.

Whether an attending gives prepared or spontaneous talks, a question that must be confronted is, How can time be preserved for such presentations? As one attending physician reported: "The problem with didactic teaching, and I've tried to do this on occasion, is that it is difficult to do because there are a certain amount of just plain ordinary problems with patients on the ward that have to be dealt with. There are times when you have something planned for presentation, and there just isn't time to do it."

Surely, uncertainties frequently crop up and make attending rounds difficult to plan. Still, as we indicated in Chapter 3, through careful allocation of time opportunities for brief talks can be protected. In particular, limiting the time spent reviewing the status of all patients by addressing only their more pressing concerns can save fifteen to twenty minutes per day (or more) that can be used for other instructional purposes.

Providing Team Members with Relevant Readings or References

Lecturing to team members is not the only way of providing them with relevant information. Another approach is to provide them with readings, such as copies of pertinent articles, references to appropriate texts, or references to particular individuals who may serve as consultants. Skeff et al. (personal communication, 22 December 1991) found that such activities are positively correlated with learners' ratings of learning outcomes. This finding is consistent with data presented by Stritter et al. (1975) and Irby (1978) regarding effective teaching across many clinical settings.

To allow for information sharing and to ensure that distributed readings actually are read, an attending may want to reserve a certain amount of time for discussion of topics covered in distributed readings or text assignments. By repeating this sort of activity too often, the attending risks turning rounds into a type of journal club. If judiciously spread out over a month, however, such discussions can provide the additional intellectual stimulation necessary to turn rounds into an optimal learning environment.

A variation on providing team members with the articles, references, or names of individuals to consult involves simply giving team members (usually students, since they have the most time) the charge of seeking information on pertinent topics and asking them to come back and educate the rest of the team. For example, Dr. Goff (whose use of probing questions was referred to earlier in this chapter) was listening to a student's case presentation and the student mentioned the fact that the patient had scarring from boils. Upon hearing this, Goff asked, "Have you read anything about boils?" When the student responded, "No," Goff quickly retorted, "Well, maybe you can inform us about them tomorrow. Why don't you go down to dermatology and find out whatever you can about her kind of boils?"

When asked about this strategy, Dr. Goff commented: "Often times . . . I'll send a student out and the next day he'll come back and give us a five minute talk on a certain area that came up in discussion. . . . It gets the student into the books again. The students get more out of it than any of us, although it's not bad for the rest of us either. . . . On many of the topics I could probably sit there and spell it all out, . . . but the students get more by having to go back and look it up."

Both medical students and residents report that this is a beneficial strategy that promotes learning and enhances team involvement. Interns, on the other hand, find such library research less appealing because of the time constraints that they face. When using this strategy, attendings should remember that their goal is to motivate learners and foster independent learning. It is very important to follow up on assignments in subsequent rounds to reinforce the learners' efforts. Similarly, attendings should be careful not to overuse the strategy, thereby dampening its appeal.

The Resident's Teaching in the Conference Room

We have explained several steps that attending physicians can take to ensure the quality of their teaching in the conference room. Two questions that we will address here are: (1) What steps can residents take to ensure high quality learning experiences during attending rounds and conference room sessions? and (2) How might residents teach in the conference room during work rounds or at other times of the day?

Residents can do quite a lot of teaching in the conference room as they conduct "sit-down" rounds or at special times set aside for teaching and learning. We have three recommendations for conference room teaching.

1. Make patient care a learning experience.
   a. Simultaneously direct the work and learning.
   b. Use probing questions to provoke thought.
   c. Point out things to learn.

2. Use illustrations and diagrams.

3. Encourage and direct reading in conjunction with or as a supplement to the attending's assigned reading.

Simultaneously Directing the Work and Learning

The most efficient way to learn patient care is to make the work experience a learning experience. This seems obvious, but it is not always easy to achieve because of the pressure of the work and fatigue. Residents, more than attendings, have the opportunity to combine work and learning. Using the "teachable moment" (see Chapter 3) to instruct is what we are suggesting. It is the residents, in fact, who make of students' rotations a learning experience or just plain scutwork. It is not surprising that students reported in a recent survey that the personal abuse they experienced came most often from residents (and part-time faculty) (Sheehan et al., 1990; Silver and Glichen, 1990). Residents can make or break the educational experience for students. If residents use opportunities to teach problem solving, question students, explain what they don't know, point out things to learn, illustrate the teaching with drawings and diagrams, and direct students' reading, then patient care can be a rich curriculum. Students recognize this potential of residents and are helpful and loyal to those residents who try to assist their learning.

There are many opportunities for residents to teach problem solving. Residents should try to be aware of these opportunities so as to make the most of them. Learning to take a history, do a physical exam, and formulate a differential diagnosis are the basic tasks of medical students. This is a problem-solving process for learners. With experience this process becomes routine recognition rather than problem solving. Experienced physicians may only have to apply a template of signs and symptoms to recognize a diagnosis instead of figuring out a problem. Every new patient presents an opportunity for students to learn the diagnostic process.

The best method to teach problem solving is to demonstrate the process and provide practice with guidance (Anderson, 1985). Residents can demonstrate the problem solving process by thinking aloud. This allows students to hear how another, more experienced learner/teacher approaches a patient problem. Practice with patients is readily available, but residents must also make the time to supervise the students and give them feedback about their data gathering and diagnostic thinking. From time to time, residents should arrange for a student to interview and examine a patient independently, without help from other persons. This is the way physicians in practice work. After the student has accomplished the task, the resident should hear the presentation of the case and discuss the student's thinking about the diagnosis.

Edwards and Marier observed a second year internal medicine resident conduct a thorough problem solving exercise with three third year students on a general medicine ward service (J. C. Edwards and R. L. Marier, "An observational study of resident teaching." In preparation).

> After lunch on a Friday afternoon, the three students reported back to the ward team. Dr. Wakeman thought a minute after the students walked up to him and asked what they should do that afternoon. Then he said, "Well, we have all the patients pretty much taken care of. Dan admitted a new patient this morning. This would be a good opportunity for you to do a thorough history and physical. I tell you what. Each of you take turns individually interviewing and examining Mrs. Williams. Do not look at her chart. Do not talk with each other about her. After you have figured out the diagnosis, then you will each present to me and we will discuss her case."
>
> Turning to the team, he said, "Don't any of you help them. They must do this on their own. This is a good way for them to learn."
>
> Turning back to the students, Dr. Wakeman said, "Let's see, one hour should be enough time for you to do that. Meet me at three o'clock in the conference room on the fourth floor west. Then I'll talk with each of you about your diagnosis."
>
> The team moved on to another floor, leaving the students to their work. At three o'clock the students showed up in the conference room. Dr. Wakeman took them into the room one at a time and, while the team listened, he had each student present the case and diagnosis to him. Then he conducted a discussion with all three students about the differential diagnoses. The exercise concluded at about half past four. One or two of the team complained about having to stay all that time on a Friday afternoon, but most thought it was a worthwhile exercise.

Another technique to teach problem solving is for the resident to pose cases from his or her own experience or to pose hypothetical cases. These cases allow the teacher to assess the student's ability to analyze and synthesize data and to formulate a diagnosis without help from charts or team members.

A method for teaching problem solving to groups is described by both Engel (1971) and Kassirer (1983). The student who presents the case is the proxy for the patient, and he or she has all the information. After the initial presentation of data, others in the group can question the proxy, but each must present the reasons for the question and relate it to a working hypothesis or diagnosis. In this manner, students are required to reveal their reasoning process and the teacher can assess and provide guidance along the way.

The following example shows a resident directing a student's presentation, using probing questions, and giving feedback.

The team gathered in the conference room just off the nurses' station at eight o'clock on Friday morning, the second day of the students' rotation. This was the students' first full day on the wards and, therefore, the first day they were expected to present patient cases. David, the resident in charge of the service, turned to Michelle, a third year student, and said, "O.K. You have the first patient, right? Let's hear it."

Michelle began, "Mrs. Hanley is a 67-year-old white female with a chief complaint of chest pain. We have to rule out MI. She had atrial fibrillation with a pacer put in ten years ago for sick sinus syndrome. She had a fibular fracture with a full leg cast on December 17th. She is scheduled for cardiac cath this morning."

David interrupted Michelle, saying, "Why don't you start with the subjective and use the same format that you use when you write a SOAP note?"

"O.K.," said Michelle. "Her vital signs are stable." She continued with the vital signs and lab values. Then she gave pertinent findings on the physical exam and current medicines, which were many. When Michelle talked about heparin, David asked her, "If her PT was bad and she was on Coumadin, how would you reverse the effects of Coumadin?"

Michelle answered, "Give her vitamin K?"

David said, "Good! Then how would you treat her if she had too much heparin on board?"

Michelle, thinking carefully, was silent for a few seconds. Then she said, "Protamine sulfate?"

David reached over and pushed his fist into Michelle's shoulder and said, "Very good!" He was obviously pleased. "What do you think the results of her cath will show?"

Michelle pondered a minute. Then she said she thought the results wouldn't show much. "The cath is being done out of consideration for her family," she said.

"That's right," David responded. "Let's go see this patient," he said.

David directed Michelle to present more information about Mrs. Hanley so that the entire team could understand the case. Then he asked probing questions of Michelle to check her knowledge and understanding of the dynamics of this particular case. Along the way, David gave positive feedback to Michelle.

Residents can give students invaluable help by pointing out things that attendings expect students to know and by teaching medical dictums.

> One day in a conference room, a team was discussing a patient with unstable angina. As they finished up the discussion, Dr. Climbers and Dr. Tipper, the two residents, exclaimed, "Hey, guys, you need to know the Killip classification for MI. Dr. Whatley is going to expect you to know that."
>
> Another day the same team was reviewing the progress of all the patients. A student was presenting Mr. Abnair, who had a large mass in his lungs with other lesions in his brain. "His blood sugar is 200 to 210; he's had a fasting one."
>
> The first year resident asked, "Do we leave him alone?"
>
> The student countered with, "Do we want to treat his blood sugar?"
>
> The first year resident said loudly and emphatically, "We don't treat numbers; we treat patients." Then he explained. "This patient has a mass that looks very much like cancer that has metastasized. The blood sugar is a little high, but is it worth using insulin? This is secondary to the cancer problem. Maybe a diet can handle the blood sugar."

Many other dictums like "We don't treat numbers; we treat patients" are handed down from residents to students. These pithy sayings capture wisdom about patient care and serve as a guide to action.

Using Illustrations and Diagrams

Illustrations and diagrams can assist learning. Residents should use chalkboards whenever they are available in conference rooms to list patient problems and draw sketches or diagrams. During work rounds, residents can make small sketches on note cards to illustrate anatomical structures and show bodily functions. (For a fuller discussion of this topic, see "Using Illustrative Devices," a section earlier in this chapter.)

Modern imaging techniques, such as Doppler studies and magnetic resonance images, enable physicians to see anatomic structures and physiologic functions inside the body that earlier generations of students could not see (Plauché and Edwards, 1988). Residents should use these images to teach students basic concepts, but they should be careful not to go beyond the depth of understanding of students. This type of teaching is best done in a conference room but is often done in hallways.

Combining the use of scientific images with the image of the actual patient at the bedside seems to be the optimal use of images in clinical teaching. That would seem to allow learners to organize mentally the scientific images around the person whom they know and treat (Edwards, 1990). This argues for conference room teaching to be closely linked in time and space to bedside teaching. Research into the mechanisms of mental processing has yet to demonstrate that as a scientific fact.

Encouraging and Directing the Students' Reading

Encouraging and directing the students' reading are valuable teaching functions. Students, of course, have an active grapevine about what books to read as well as much other "survival" information. Direction form the resident in charge of the service, however, is usually welcomed.

On the first day of an Internal Medicine rotation for third year students, Dr. Climbers asked the students, "Did they recommend to you in the orientation any manuals, like SCUT Monkcy or the Washington University manual?"

The students said, "No."

"Well, don't go out and buy Cecil's. I can recommend a couple of good books. *The Clinician's Pocket Guide: The Scut Monkey,* by Lange. Also the Washington University manual on patient management. Get one book and stick with it. Don't go book hopping. I'll give you supplemental papers and articles."

The Benefit of a Private Location

Modern teaching hospitals are busy places in which physicians are always in demand. The medical services' conference room provides a quiet sanctuary where teaching can be done with decreased fear of being interrupted and decreased concern about being overheard. Too much time in the conference room can put the team out of touch with patients and other health care personnel not participating in the conference room sessions. However, judicious use of the conference room is a powerful stimulus to learning that should be part of any teaching physician's instructional repertoire.

CHAPTER FIVE

Teaching at the Bedside

After the conference room presentations, Dr. Jeffries, an oncologist, went to the new patients' bedsides with the three medical students, the intern who had been on call the previous evening, and the resident. After politely introducing himself and the accompanying team members, Dr. Jeffries began interviewing the first patient, Mr. Wolfe. Jeffries soon discovered that Mr. Wolfe had initially visited his local doctor because of repeated bouts of tiredness early in the day. This piece of information had not been included in the intern's conference room presentation. The intern had reported that Mr. Wolfe had gone to his doctor merely to have a periodic check-up. Further questioning revealed that Mr. Wolfe had also been concerned about a small amount of weight loss, a point also missed by the intern.

While doing a partial physical examination, Dr. Jeffries demonstrated to the accompanying team members how to find the lymph nodes. Jeffries quietly explained to the team members what he felt as his hands searched for the nodes. He directed the team's attention to a small node near Mr. Wolfe's elbow which had not been reported by the intern in the conference room presentation. Dr. Jeffries then pointed out deep iliac nodes below the stomach which were also missed by the intern. Jeffries explicitly demonstrated how to find the iliac nodes and then had the intern and the students find them also.

Although he was quite gentle throughout his methodical examination, Dr. Jeffries apologized to Mr. Wolfe for "all of the poking," explaining that it was necessary to obtain a complete assessment of Mr. Wolfe's current condition and to put together the best possible treatment plan.

The Attending Physician's Bedside Teaching

The scene described above illustrates one of the most delicate aspects of clinical instruction—bedside teaching. The challenge of simultaneously addressing the patient's emotional needs and the team's learning needs demands sensitivity, tact, knowledge, instructional skill, and good management of time. Bedside teaching is often a hit or miss affair. When things go well, as in the above case with Dr. Jeffries, there is a great discovery and everyone present is excited and engaged. However, often no great discovery is uncovered and the team exhibits only passive involvement. Thus, it is incumbent upon the attending physician to engage the team creatively whenever possible.

Since bedside teaching serves several purposes, various opportunities for engaging the team exist. In addition to uncovering new findings, bedside visits allow attending physicians to confirm and agree on management of routine cases, provide assistance in complicated cases, assess team members' abilities, and provide patients with new information or education. By keeping their objectives flexible, attendings can invite team involvement in each of these areas. This may require making assignments for people to observe certain portions of the interaction that will transpire or assigning certain individuals to do parts of the history or physical exam. To promote high-quality bedside teaching, we also offer the following recommendations.

1. Use the patient for effective teaching whenever possible. However, be conscious of the time demands placed on team members. Make bedside visits concise. Rather than requiring all team members to visit all patients during rounds, consider having team members visit only their own patients and specific patients from whom they might learn a great deal.

2. Use the hallway efficiently. Limit the time spent on patient presentations and discussions in the hallway, and minimize probing questions. If lengthy follow-up discussions are required, move to the conference room.

3. Generally, reserve case presentations for the conference room; but if requiring presentations at the bedside, take precautions to avoid causing patients distress.

4. Make bedside teaching explicit. When possible, alert team members beforehand to skills that will be demonstrated at

the bedside. Whether or not forewarning is possible, address bedside interactions in follow-up discussions.

5. Focus on teaching both physical skills (e.g., conducting a physical exam) and interpersonal skills (e.g., eliciting an accurate history or addressing the patient's personal needs).

6. When possible, observe team members as they perform the physical and interpersonal skills that you have demonstrated and give them feedback on their performances.

Using the Patient for Teaching

William Osler, the bedside teacher par excellence, used patients as the primary vehicle for his teaching. The Oslerian teaching model became a standard for medical faculty that still endures (Linfors and Neelon, 1980). As Osler said, there should be "no teaching without a patient for a text, and the best teaching is that taught by the patient himself" (Osler, 1903).

Why is bedside, patient-centered teaching so effective? Evidence suggests that we develop mental images when engaging in tasks involving spatial or visual information (Gagne, 1985). Since patients' bodies convey such information, students and house staff naturally form strong images of patients. Also, we learn and remember information by associating ideas in memory networks (Wittrock, 1986). Patient-centered teaching enables trainees to remember patients and to associate new information with those patients, thereby establishing concentrated, focused memory networks (Plauché and Edwards, 1988).

Medical tradition and recent psychologic research, then, both point to patient-centered teaching as an effective way to learn medicine. Attending physicians would do well to rely on patients whenever possible in their teaching. Interviewing and physical diagnosis are taught best with the patient present. Much of the teaching of clinical procedures can be done with patients. Professional reading can center around the patients being cared for by the team. Learning that takes place at the patient's side is likely to be processed deeply and associated with previous learning in the memory network and to be readily available for future clinical use.

In spite of the inherent advantages of patient-centered teaching, some attending physicians conduct rounds solely in the conference room, some engage in only a ritual tour of their patients' bedsides without initiating any real teaching efforts, and most divide their teaching efforts between the conference room and the bedside, with the conference room receiving the major allocation of time (Shankel and Mazzaferri, 1986; Weinholtz, 1981). Responding to these trends, Linfors and Neelon (1980) argued for abandoning the conference room completely in favor of bedside rounds. We, on the other hand, advocate judiciously using both the bedside and the conference room, drawing on the advantages of both settings as conditions warrant.

When selecting patients for teaching, attending physicians must remember that interns at many teaching hospitals tour the patients' bedsides during morning work rounds, and interns at all teaching hospitals have pressing demands of patient care throughout the day. Consequently, they often become impatient with bedside teaching directed specifically to medical students and with bedside visits involving little teaching, such as occasions when attendings conduct lengthy patient interviews yielding no pertinent new information. Under such circumstances the interns simply feel that their time could be better spent elsewhere (Weinholtz, 1981).

Attendings can address this legitimate frustration by conferring with the resident and selectively choosing the patients that they require interns to visit during attending rounds. Although medical students may also develop negative attitudes about seeing all patients, they will probably benefit from accompanying the attending physician to see every patient that he or she visits. Interns, however, need only visit their own patients and particular patients from whom they might learn a great deal. Because residents are responsible for all patients, it follows that they should visit all the patients that the attending visits during rounds.

Dr. Waitzman, a cardiologist, illustrates effective bedside instruction on a patient selected to teach the entire team (Weinholtz, 1981).

> One day he arranged for a multiple-auscultation machine to be on his service. By hooking up every member of the team, Waitzman was able to review simultaneously for six learners (three students, two interns, and the resident) the different heart sounds associated with different chest areas of a patient. While doing so he illustrated the pulsating in the patient's chest by quickly raising and lowering

his pen, which he rested on the auscultation machine. The pen thus resembled a gauge fluctuating rhythmically with the patient's heart beat. Throughout, Dr. Waitzman managed to keep the patient at ease by engaging him in good-humored conversation.

After leaving the patient's room, a student quietly commented, "This was a very good thing to listen to. He was my patient and I really got a lot out of listening."

In an interview a week later, the service resident offered: "Dr. Waitzman's physical exam teaching is great. He does more of it and is better at it than any I have seen. The effort that he puts in! For example, he got those earphones up here for us and enabled everybody to listen!"

Clearly, when the attending has something to offer at the bedside, team members at all levels will appreciate it. To ensure such focused teaching efforts, Schwenk and Whitman (1987) argued for separating more formalized bedside teaching from attending round teaching by scheduling selected patients at distinct times for "demonstrating physical findings, interviewing a particularly difficult patient, or teaching a specific procedure." While there is obvious merit to this suggestion, the unique demands of a particular service and the teaching strengths of the individual attending physician will always interact to determine what approaches to bedside teaching are both feasible and desirable.

Teaching in the Hallway

Attending physicians generally spend more than 20 percent of their rounding time in hallways (Schor and Grayson, 1984; Weinholtz et al., 1986a). Although little has been written about hallways as teaching settings, strong negative correlations between time spent on teaching activities in hallways and team members' ratings of teaching effectiveness have been reported (Weinholtz et al., 1986a). These negative correlations were especially pronounced when the relationship between time spent asking probing questions (i.e., those questions initiated for instructional purposes) and team members' ratings were examined.

There are several reasons why hallways may not be optimal teaching settings. First, they contain many distractions that divert team members' attention. Second, hallways are public places where team members may feel uneasy about being challenged and patients' rights to privacy may be compromised. Third, team members view a grand tour of the patients' rooms via hallways as redundant with morning work rounds. Fourth, team members often do not like to stand if they think that they could just as easily be sitting.

In spite of these inherent instructional obstacles, it is obvious that hallways cannot be avoided completely. Any time the attending wants to take the team to the bedside, a hallway must be navigated. The major concern regarding hallways seems to be judicious use of time. It seems undesirable to engage in lengthy hallway discussions of cases not just because it is tiring and distracting for team members but also because hallway discussions potentially involve disclosing confidential information within earshot of visitors, personnel, and patients passing through the hallway. Furthermore, probing questions used to provoke thought or assess team members' understanding seem better suited for the reflective environment of the conference room than for hallways, where background noise and interruptions may fluster team members. Thus, it seems wiser to initiate most instructional efforts in the conference room or at the bedside, reserving the hallway primarily as the conduit between the two or as the location for brief, discrete follow-up commentaries after patient encounters. Such commentaries can focus on specific teaching points or offer capsule summaries of principles to be retained from patient visits.

Listening to Case Presentations

Very little research has specifically addressed the merits and problems associated with having students and house staff give oral case presentations at the bedside. A controlled study examining the effects of conference room and bedside presentations on patients and team members is currently in process at Hennepin County Hospital in Minneapolis, Minnesota, under the direction of Michael Belzer, M.D. Until the results of this study are available, findings from descriptive studies must guide our recommendations.

Linfors and Neelon (1980) cited a survey of fifty patients in a journal article strongly advocating bedside rounds. The survey ascertained the patients' "responses to the bedside presentation of their case histories." Ninety-four percent of the patients indicated that they were pleased with their bedside sessions. One indicated that any discussion was inappropriate. Ninety-four percent believed that such rounds should continue, and ninety percent did not wish to change any aspect. On the other hand, thirty-four percent reported that the presentations did not help them better understand their problems, and thirty-six percent reported that they were not properly forewarned. The authors viewed their findings as consistent with Romano's (1941) finding that "ward rounds teaching, when conducted tactfully and sympathetically, is not a traumatic emotional experience to patients but educates and reassures them."

We believe that it is indeed possible to conduct bedside case presentations in a manner that is time efficient, educational, and reassuring to patients. However, given the anxiety reported by several of Romano's (1941) patients, as well as the finding that the time spent by attending physicians listening to patient presentations and discussions at the bedside was significantly and negatively correlated with teaching-effectiveness ratings by medical students and interns (Weinholtz et al., 1986a), we advise restraint regarding the use of bedside case presentations. This more recent study may suffer from an uncontrolled bias as it was conducted in a teaching hospital where case presentations are typically given in the conference room. Similar correlational studies in hospitals where there is a long tradition of bedside presentations have not yet been conducted. In the absence of such data, it seems prudent to reserve presentations for the conference room except when there seems to be clear instructional benefit and no chance of harm to the patient. However, if using bedside case presentations, an attending physician should certainly follow the few recommendations offered by Linfors and Neelon. Their patients gave the following suggestions for the attending physician.

1. Provide the patient with advance notice of bedside rounds.

2. Introduce himself or herself and clearly state the purpose of the bedside rounds.

3. Translate technical terms for the patient.

4. Limit the length of time at the bedside so as not to tire the patient.

Indeed, these are worthwhile recommendations to follow whenever the team visits the bedside. We also believe in going a step further; if the patient expresses serious reservations concerning bedside rounds, the attending should comply with the patient's wishes. Certainly, alternatives to taking a large entourage to the bedside do exist. As an attending expressed: "I don't like to do bedside teaching with a large audience because it is disrespectful to the patient. I view myself as a somewhat private person and I like to have that privacy protected. I feel that patients deserve the same. They should be able to relate to their physician without having a whole entourage present. So, what I often do is come back after dinner, grab the student and intern on call, and go to see the patients."

Teaching Explicitly

Attendings who teach at the bedside often report that they attempt to model the clinical skills displayed by their favorite attendings from medical school or residency training. However, these attendings rarely make their role modeling explicit. Instead, they rely on the students and house staff to infer for themselves lessons based on what they observe (Schor and Grayson, 1984; Weinholtz, 1981).

Unfortunately, team members may miss subtle but important aspects of bedside demonstrations if their attention is not directed specifically to those aspects by their clinical instructors (Stritter and Flair, 1980). To minimize this sort of slippage, attendings can alert team members to their intentions before entering the patient's room or, if appropriate, at the patient's bedside itself. Residents may also be aware of specific points while the attending is teaching and may alert the other team members to the attendings' actions and words. Such announcements will help to focus the team members' attention on what they are supposed to observe, thereby optimizing their ability to ask questions, integrate their observations with prior knowledge, and retain what they have learned. Brief follow-up discussions led by the attending physician can be used to draw the team members' attention to aspects of the patient interaction when no prior warning was possible. Follow-up discussions can also be used to answer team members' questions, to place the bedside demonstration in its appropriate context, and to reinforce the points that the attending wants the team members to retain.

The following illustration shows how an attending physician used a bedside encounter to reinforce explicitly an important clinical point associated with eliciting an accurate patient history.

During rounds Dr. Goff, who had an exceptional rapport with her team, repeatedly reminded the group to be alert for drug reactions in patients. For example, on her first day on the services she told the team that "for any illness" they "should think drugs first!" Goff explained that "a patient may become hypersensitive to any drug; Goody Powder, Anacin, anything!" Two days later she reinforced the point in the conference room during the first of two student presentations. After the student's presentation of the patient's history, Dr. Goff humorously interrupted before the student could proceed with the review of systems, exclaiming, "Whoa! You forgot the most important ingredient in the history. You forgot to summarize what kind of drugs that he is on."

Frank, the student, responded, "No drugs."

"How about Goody Powder or laxatives? Can laxatives cause you any trouble?"

Frank acknowledged, "Laxatives could cause you trouble if you took a load of them." He also indicated that he was unsure whether or not his patient was taking laxatives.

Following Frank's presentation, another student, Justine, presented the case of Mrs. Densen, a patient suffering from an ulcer. Since Justine was very well organized, Dr. Goff let her proceed without interruption until she reviewed Mrs. Densen's medicines. After Justine mentioned Bufferin, Goff asked, "How often does she take Bufferin?"

"Only occasionally for chronic headaches, but I didn't nail her down to exactly how many."

Later in the morning, while at Mrs. Densen's bedside eliciting her own brief history, Dr. Goff specifically asked her how many Bufferin or Anacin she normally took in a day. Mrs. Densen responded that she averaged six Anacin per day for her headaches.

In the hallway, after leaving Mrs. Densen's room, Dr. Goff turned to Justine and good-naturedly scolded, "Six Anacin a day. You didn't tell me that."

Somewhat taken a back, Justine collegially jousted, "Well, she told me that it was only occasional."

"If she admits to as many as six," Goff explained, "she may well be taking as many as eight or ten. And that could be the reason behind her ulcer."

The incident just described was brief; the bedside encounter with Mrs. Densen took only seven or eight minutes, and the critical question regarding Anacin took just a few seconds. However, Dr. Goff exhibited incisive bedside teaching. She had established her concern about drugs early in the month. She reinforced her point about drugs twice in the conference room before visiting Mrs. Densen. She explicitly modeled for the team how to elicit a specific response from the patient. Finally, she immediately followed up on the implications of the new information with the student and the rest of the team.

Of course, one might have asked even more of Dr. Goff. She might have alerted Justine and the rest of the team immediately before entering Mrs. Densen's room that she was going to ask the question regarding drugs. She also might have expanded the discussion following the visit to Mrs. Densen's room to include the merits and problems of particular questioning strategies. Such additional efforts would have been beneficial. Still, Dr. Goff's teaching was both efficient and valuable to the team.

Frank was the student Dr. Goff challenged regarding awareness of patients' medicines before Justine's presentation. His reaction to the incident with Mrs. Densen tells a great deal. Immediately after rounds, Frank exclaimed: "Dr. Goff is just super. . . . Justine's case had a beautiful illustration of the point about drugs that she made during my presentation. . . . There is just so much that you have to learn that it is really important for the attending to pick out the things that are central and to drive them home again and again. Up until now I have never really paid the attention that I should to what kind of drugs a patient is on. Dr. Goff has driven that point home, and I'll be much more sensitive in the future."

A further point must be made. Dr. Goff's challenge of Justine could be viewed as an unnecessary public humiliation. Indeed, it might have been if not delivered by an attending physician with Dr. Goff's deft social skills. Justine clearly enjoyed her interactions with Dr. Goff and compared her favorably to other attendings with whom she had worked. Also, Justine was a fourth year student doing an elective in internal medicine. She was more confident than the other students and appeared to handle challenges well. As she later indicated, "you . . . learn not to take it too seriously." Such confidence is less typical among many third year students, who might have to be confronted in a more discrete manner.

Teaching Physical and Interpersonal Skills

The bedside is ideally suited for modeling and teaching both physical skills, such as the physical examination, and interpersonal skills, such as eliciting a history or addressing the patient's personal needs. Attendings rarely conduct complete physical examinations during rounds because of the redundancy with the students' and the house staff's earlier physical exams. However, brief partial exams focusing on key findings pertinent to patients' diagnoses are especially well suited for rounds. By conducting such exams, the attending can confirm the presence of particular symptoms, refute their presence, or discover additional findings missed by the student, intern, or resident. These partial physicals at the bedside provide excellent teaching opportunities. An illustration of one such opportunity was presented at the beginning of this chapter where Dr. Jeffries was described demonstrating to team members how to find various types of nodes and allowing the team members to find the nodes for themselves.

Another physician who was observed in the same study (Weinholtz, 1981) and was particularly adept at teaching physical exam skills was Dr. Goff, a gastroenterologist.

> Recognizing the need to put her patients at ease before the physical, she always gently joked with patients a bit before examining them. While giving a partial examination, Dr. Goff regularly emphasized to team members commonsense approaches to diagnosis that can give the physician important insights before laboratory test results can be obtained. For example, while examining one patient, she told the team that hematocrit levels can be estimated by looking at the patient's fingernails and eyelids. Then, while holding the patient's hand at an angle where she and the rest of the team could clearly view the fingernails, Goff ventured a guess of the patient's hematocrit level. A subsequent check of the lab tests showed that she was right. Her students all registered looks indicating that they were clearly impressed.
>
> Later, when asked about her priorities for bedside teaching, Dr. Goff responded: "Well, meeting the patients is number one. . . .

Also, I like to home in on their primary problems through the history and the physical exam. I've already heard the presentation in the conference room, but I like to create a situation where the house staff and the students can see in a quick way how I would attack the problem. I like to spend a little time with them going over specific physical findings, so they can see where I go, and what I do. Generally, that's about all that you have time for if you have two or more new patients."

Her approach made a clear impression on students. One afternoon following rounds, two students, Wilma and Frank, discussed what they had learned earlier in the day.

"I learned a lot of physical diagnosis!" commented Wilma. "You know the little pustules around her eye. I saw them before, but I never paid any attention to them. Dr. Goff manages to point out all of the little things that you read about in the books but then manage to forget. I also was impressed with the way she laid hands on her. I mean she really felt comfortable touching her. That just wasn't the case with the last attending."

"But the last attending did physical exams on the patients," interjected Frank.

"Yes, but it wasn't the same," offered Wilma. "It was rigid and formal. This was much more natural, and she did it in a way that the patient didn't mind."

"Yeah, you could see how comfortable Dr. Goff made her feel," Frank agreed.

As this illustration shows, in addition to being a site for teaching physical examination skills, the bedside is also particularly well suited for modeling appropriate interactions with patients. These interactions may include methods of eliciting history, patient education techniques, or ways of showing attentiveness to patients' personal needs. Although all of these interactions are important aspects of a physician's education, many attendings tend to underemphasize them during rounds (Adams et al., 1964; Reichsman et al., 1964; Payson and Barchas, 1965; Weinholtz, 1981). Dawson and Patel (1983) reported that students with high patient contact over a clinical rotation showed a significant increase in their interpersonal skills during patient interactions. Optimally, the frequently recurring opportunities for teaching such skills will be seized and converted by attendings into explicit learning experiences.

The previous section on "explicit teaching" contained an illustration of how an attending physician used a bedside encounter to teach the elicitation of a history. Here we present further illustrations indicating how attendings might draw on bedside situations to teach the importance of meeting patients' personal needs.

> On his first day in attending rounds, Dr. O'Leary alerted his team, while in the conference room, that "we are terribly deficient in meeting the total needs of our patients. Too often we just approach our patients' care through giving pills and inserting tubes. There is far more than that."
>
> Later, O'Leary provided the team with several suggestions regarding ways they could provide interpersonal support for patients on the service. He chastised an intern, and the team in general, for making only half-hearted efforts in this direction for Mr. Fairley, a paraplegic pulmonary patient with a two-year history of severe depression. Dr. O'Leary was particularly distressed that the team had apparently written Mr. Fairley off as a case for the social workers and psychiatric consult team. O'Leary challenged the team to use the occasion and meet Mr. Fairley's needs for interaction with concerned individuals. He told them that they would be failing in their responsibilities as physicians if they compartmentalized patient care by turning over all the psychosocial aspects to others.
>
> Outside of rounds, Mr. Fairley's intern and the service resident reported that they were touched by Dr. O'Leary's concern for Mr. Fairley but that Dr. O'Leary was probably overstating his point. Mr. Fairley's lung disease was manageable, but various medical services and social work teams had been attempting to help with his depression for a long time without any results. The house staff saw little hope for any improvement in Mr. Fairley, who continued to lie unresponsive in a dark room during his stay on their service.
>
> No single bedside visit by Dr. O'Leary appeared to trigger a change in Mr. Fairley, but day in and day out O'Leary was observed by team members interacting with Mr. Fairley in a pleasant, concerned fashion. They noted that O'Leary frequently stopped by Mr. Fairley's room during other times of day after rounds were completed.
>
> One day in the conference room at the beginning of rounds, Dr. O'Leary remarked: "Incidentally, yesterday I saw something that opened my heart. Mr. Fairley was smiling, and do you know why?

It was because a pretty young woman (a hospital volunteer) was playing chess with him. This indicates to me that to help him we really don't have to do all that much. . . . As soon as a member of his family comes, call me, even if I am at home. I will be glad to come up so that we can have a conference."

Within a few days, Dr. O'Leary himself was regularly scheduling chess games with Mr. Fairley. By the end of two weeks a dramatic change had occurred. Mr. Fairley, whom team members had previously avoided, became one of the most popular patients on the service. Commenting on the turn-around, one of the residents stated: "If there is one thing that I will never forget in my medical career, it is the change that Dr. O'Leary helped to bring about in Bill Fairley. We used to just walk by there in the morning and stick our heads in the door to say, 'Hey, Bill, are you going to recreation therapy today?' It took Dr. O'Leary to show us that we had to give him more than that.

"Dr. O'Leary has a very deep concern for people's total well-being: physical, emotional, psychologic, and spiritual. It is something that you may have or can develop, but it can't be taught except by example. Dr. O'Leary makes you realize that here is a man who is concerned about something, that you are not as concerned as he is, and that maybe you ought to be."

Obviously, the case of Dr. O'Leary and Mr. Fairley is a particularly dramatic one that is not easily replicated. Still, as Siegel (1986) pointed out, opportunities to engage patients in the challenge of healing themselves both physically and emotionally occur all the time on medical services. These opportunities, even if far less dramatic than that provided by Mr. Fairley, provide attending physicians with valuable occasions for teaching how to meet patients' psychosocial needs.

On a daily basis, with many or all patients, attendings can model several very simple but important behaviors demonstrating their concerns for patients' needs. For example, before leaving his patients' bedsides, Dr. O'Leary always asked the patients and any family members who might be present if they had any questions for him. His invitation for questions was always open-ended and offered in such a way as to let the patients and family drive the discussion.

Like Dr. O'Leary, another physician observed in the same study, Dr. Waitzman, had a knack for developing a strong rapport with patients. Referring to his practice of sitting down next to his patients while talking to them, Dr. Waitzman commented: "I do that on purpose, not just because it is more comfortable, but because there is something about sitting down with some-body . . . that helps you to enter a more empathetic relationship. It enables you to convey that the patient is your main object of concern, which he is."

Many team members working with both Dr. Waitzman and Dr. O'Leary sensed the empathy that the attendings had for their patients, admired the concern that the attendings were able to demonstrate, and wished to emulate the attendings' behaviors. However, in spite of being exceptional role models, Dr. O'Leary and Dr. Waitzman missed many opportunities to reinforce in their students an awareness of specific ways of interacting with patients. As is the case with many people who are at ease and supportive in demanding interpersonal situations, the attend-ings' own behaviors had become second nature to them. Their behaviors were reflexive and not the sorts of thing that they con-sciously examined. Thus, they often were not inclined to return to the hallway or move to the conference room to discuss with team members how they had interacted with patients during what they considered to be routine situations. Some good teach-ing opportunities for both students and house staff were lost.

As we have previously indicated, bedside teaching is op-timized through explicit follow-up discussion. Follow-up dis-cussions would probably be burdensome if conducted too often but are clearly justifiable several times throughout the course of a month. Attendings hoping to maximize the teaching influence of personal interactions with patients should reflect on their own ways of dealing with patients, isolate those behaviors that they consider to be most effective, and raise the topic of these behav-iors for explicit discussion with team members at appropriate times. In this way, these important interpersonal issues can be-come a more formal part of the clinical curriculum.

Observing Performances and Providing Feedback

Although it is important for attendings to model skills at the bedside and discuss these skills with team members, modeling and discussion are insufficient to ensure that learning is occur-ring on the part of either students or house staff. Ideally, attend-ings must take the additional steps of observing team members performing bedside skills and providing the team members with feedback regarding their performances. Several studies documented that such bedside observations with accompanying feedback are too rarely provided team members (Reichsman et al., 1964; Payson and Barchas, 1965; Daggett, 1977; Weinholtz, 1981; Schor and Grayson, 1984).

Obviously, daily demands intrude on an attending's opportunities to observe team members at the bedside. However, there is reason to believe that such opportunities can be provided if conscious effort is made. Hinz (1966) evaluated both the effects and the costs of having attending physicians directly observe and evaluate medical students' clinical skills. He found that direct observation was a valuable teaching device because of the specific feedback that it permitted. He also reported that direct observation was well accepted by students, patients, and faculty. However, the faculty did view the technique as particularly costly of their time. Further evidence of the value of demonstrating physical exam skills followed by observing team members searching for physical findings was reported by Weinholtz et al. (1986a), who cited positive correlations between such activities and team members' rating of attending physicians' teaching effectiveness.

Engel (1971) reported an interesting technique that he used with medical students in a wide variety of inpatient and outpatient services. The approach involves observing a brief patient interview as a springboard for both feedback and medical problem-solving discussions. It requires using both the bedside and the conference room and allows team members other than the attending physician the opportunity to comment on the interviewer's performance.

> The exercise begins at the bedside with an interview that is arbitrarily terminated within 15 to 20 minutes, the patient being told that time has run out but that the group or the student assigned to him will return later. In the first few sessions the instructor interviews. Thereafter, these interviews are conducted by a student, though to emphasize points of technic, the instructor may also interview briefly after the student has finished. The group then retires to the classroom, where the exercise proceeds in the following sequence.
>
> Discussion begins with an evaluation of the interview technic

whether performed by the instructor or the student. The instructor may point out aspects of his own interview strategy or identify difficulties he had with the patient. The student who interviewed is first asked to evaluate his own performance, not omitting reference to his own ease or discomfort, and his feelings about the patient. His fellow students are also asked to comment on his performance, after which the instructor makes his evaluation. The emphasis at this time is on technic rather than on content, which will be considered later in the exercise.

Students are next asked to describe the patient, including his general appearance, obvious physical signs, degree of illness, his behavior and his relation with the interviewer, as well as features of his hospital room, including the presence of flowers, cards, reading material, or visitors.

The students are then required to characterize the patient in one or two sentences in terms of age, sex, occupation, marital status, family status, ethnic background, religion and other relevant identifying information such as blindness, established diabetes and status as welfare recipient or war veteran. This procedure is used to emphasize the value of such information in establishing the uniqueness of the patient as an individual and in defining his place in the social matrix. Furthermore, it immediately calls attention to obvious and important omissions in the course of the interview. . . .

The student who interviewed is now called upon to summarize the information revealed during his 15-minute interview. In the course of his effort to construct a coherent account not only will glaring omissions in the interview be quickly exposed but also other students may well disagree in substance and emphasis about what the patient reported. All this provides the instructor with an opportunity to demonstrate how clinical data may be organized and its reliability assayed. (Engel, 1971, p. 21–22)

Such sessions can stand alone or can be expanded into discussions focusing on developing and testing clinical hypotheses. Also, observations of the physical examination might be included. Whatever options are chosen, it is the observation of the patient encounter that launches the discussion and provides the interviewing student and the other participants with a valuable learning experience. Finally, while Engel emphasized the value of this approach with medical students, adaptations for use with house staff should not be ruled out. For example, patients with particularly complex histories or subtle physical symptoms may well provide interns' or residents' with substantial data-collection challenges, enabling them to benefit greatly from observation and feedback by the attending and other members of the team.

Obviously, good teaching such as this does not come without some costs. If opportunities for observation and feedback are to be provided during rounds, the attending may have to spend additional time on the medical service visiting patients who could not be seen during the regular rounds. On the other hand, if an attending is intent on a large number of patient visits during rounds, additional blocks of time will have to be reserved for providing team members with observation and feedback.

The Resident's Bedside Teaching

Residents can assist attending physicians with bedside teaching during attending rounds. They can also do substantial amounts of bedside teaching during work rounds and at other times of the day. During attending rounds, a resident can

1. prompt students to give answers and responses,
2. elaborate on what the attending is explaining or demonstrating, and
3. elicit teaching from the attending.

During work rounds and at other times of the day, the resident can go to the bedside to

4. reinforce or correct the attending's teaching,
5. teach clinical procedures, or
6. teach history-taking and physical examination skills.

Prompting Students to Give Answers and Responses

Students may need to be prompted on rounds with the attending, particularly at the patient's bedside. Because the communication process is complicated with both the patient and the attending present, students frequently need help remembering what to say to whom and when to say it. Residents can diplomatically give cues. However, residents should not give cues to camouflage a student' deficiencies. Attendings need to see for themselves each team member's performance and work intellectually with each member (Edwards and Marier, 1988).

Dr. Climber, a second year medicine resident, said about students' information base: "It's in there, but you have to get them pointed in a certain direction. Once you point them in a certain direction, the light comes on. Then they can answer the question and explain it. I'm the students' advocate. Lots of times attendings ask questions inappropriate for students. For example, that question on rounds today about interpreting the EKG. That was too advanced for their level of education. So I prompted them. That handled the situation."

Elaborating on the Instruction by the Attending Physician

Sometimes during attending rounds, the resident can assist the attending's teaching by elaborating on what the attending is explaining or demonstrating. Attendings who are expert may fail to explain all of the intermediate steps in logic of a diagnosis or treatment plan or may fail to articulate the major points of a physical demonstration. Residents, who are closer in level of learning to students, may recognize and explain these points (Steward and Feltovich, 1988). The following example illustrates.

After attending rounds one morning, Dr. Climber, the resident in charge of the service, took the students aside and said to them, "I'm not sure you understood Dr. Whatley's question about EKGs. We don't really expect you at your level of training to be able to interpret EKGs skillfully. But you should know the basics about EKGs. So let's go over things like rate, rhythm, axis, hypertrophy, ischemia, and infarction. This will be a review of the basics for you."

Eliciting Teaching from the Attending Physician

Some attending physicians do not provide much teaching. Residents can try to elicit teaching whenever a learning opportunity arises but is not acted on by the attending. Asking questions of the attending is the best way to approach this delicate task. The resident in charge can consider himself or herself a coteacher in these circumstances and can question other team members and offer explanations to create an adequate learning experience during attending rounds.

Reinforcing or Correcting the Attending Physician's Teaching

Ordinarily the resident can reinforce the attending's bedside teaching after rounds. The resident can check for understanding among the team members about the important points that emerged on rounds. Explanations may have to be repeated or additional information may be needed.

Occasionally, an attending physician sets a bad example at the bedside. When this happens, it usually involves interpersonal relations with a patient or family. When that is clearly the case, the resident in charge, in private conference with the team away from the patient, may diplomatically and nonjudgmentally point out the example and mention or develop with the group a better way to handle the situation. However, residents should not use their near-peer influence with interns and students to mitigate the attending's role, integrity, or competence. The resident in the situation described below showed proper discretion.

> As the attending, Dr. Bauer, and his ward team approached a patient's room on rounds one afternoon, the third year resident, Dr. Perkins, turned to him and said softly, "You will be nice to Mr. Williams today, won't you? He needs your care." When questioned later about this interchange, Dr. Perkins explained that on the previous day Dr. Bauer had been rude to Mr. Williams, an indigent alcoholic with multiple medical problems. She explained that Dr. Bauer, a GI specialist, was well known among the staff for his prejudice against alcoholics. Dr. Perkins explained that she had intervened on behalf of the patient and the students because she thought that rude behavior to patients set a poor example for students.

Teaching Clinical Procedures

Students learn many clinical procedures from interns and residents, and it is important for residents to teach procedures thoroughly. Much research in psychology, movement science, and the military has documented an effective method for teaching physical skills. This method involves breaking the procedure down into a series of small steps, explaining and demonstrating the steps in sequence, and then giving supervised practice with feedback (Foley and Smilansky, 1980). If the resident can anticipate problems and prepare the student to handle these before starting the procedure, the learning will go more smoothly. Without a detailed explanation of the steps or a demonstration, students cannot learn to perform a procedure correctly. Time spent in teaching the steps explicitly is worthwhile.

The following illustration indicates how a resident can effectively teach a clinical procedure.

> Dr. Perkins and the three students were at the bedside of Mrs. Mary Bowman, an elderly patient with renal failure, organic brain syndrome, and hypertension. Dr. Perkins had greeted Mrs. Bowman's niece, who was standing near the bed with her hand gently held on Mrs. Bowman's forehead. Dr. Perkins said to the students, "These are work rounds. Get the gloves." After putting on gloves, she began to probe the left groin, looking for an artery. After much searching on the left and right groin, Dr. Perkins finally felt an artery. Parting the folds of skin with her right hand, she turned to the students and asked, "Do you know how to do a femoral stick?"
>
> Jim answered, "You palpate the femoral artery below the inguinal ligament and go 1 centimeter medial to the pulsating artery."
>
> Perkins said, "Yes." Then she sterilized the whole area. She turned to Tom who was standing closest to her and directed the rest of the instructions to him. "Palpate the artery with your left hand and, using the right hand, stick 1 centimeter medially to your finger, holding the syringe perpendicular to the body. As soon as you pierce the skin, pull up on the plunger with your right thumb, as you push the syringe deeper. As soon as you hit the vein, pull the plunger with your left hand. If you go deeper than the vein should be before you get any blood, pull out slowly until you get some blood."
>
> Turning her head toward Mrs. Bowman, she said, "Mrs. Bowman, there's going to be a big stick." Mrs. Bowman started moaning softly.
>
> Tom began to repeat the verbal instructions aloud to make sure he had it in memory. When he finished, Dr. Perkins pointed to the artery with her finger. She allowed Tom to palpate the artery. She pointed to the spot to stick. He stuck the needle in, pulled up on the plunger with his right thumb, and proceeded to go deeper. As soon as he hit the vein, he reached with his left hand to pull on the plunger and got only a couple of milliliters of blood before losing the vein. Dr. Perkins told him to go a little deeper while maintaining

suction. After having done that, she told him to pull back some. Tom tried, but he couldn't find the vein again. Dr. Perkins got a new syringe and repeated the procedure.

Dr. Perkins asked Jim to apply pressure to the site for five minutes to prevent bleeding.

When Tom finished transferring the blood, he disposed of the materials, and they all went to wash their hands. As the entire team walked down the hall, Tom thanked Dr. Perkins. She put her hand on his shoulder briefly and said, "You'll do a few more before you leave here, and then you'll be an expert!"

Dr. Perkins gave a detailed verbal explanation of each step in the procedure. She also prepared Tom for the difficulty he actually encountered in drawing the blood. This helped him to deal with the difficulty and also let him know that difficulty was common. Tom verbalized the steps after Dr. Perkins had but before he tried the procedure. Not all students will do this; the resident should ask the student to repeat the instructions before beginning.

Teaching History Taking, Physical Examination, Differential Diagnosis, and Problem Solving

Residents encounter many opportunities to go to the bedside and teach students history taking, physical examination, and problem solving, particularly the differential diagnosis. The circumstances of an extended time period and the admission of new patients combine to make this an excellent opportunity to teach the full front-end process of inpatient care. Since fatigue mitigates against this teaching opportunity, residents must schedule effectively to teach when fatigue is low and when the team can be intellectually productive.

The resident in charge should assign each new patient to a student and intern or resident. Students should be given the responsibility to interview and examine patients independently. Then they should be required to present to the resident their findings, impression, and differential diagnosis. Only in this way will they learn the skills that practicing physicians must possess.

The following illustration shows a resident effectively teaching physical diagnosis during morning work rounds.

Dr. Perkins and the three students arrived at Mrs. Blackmore's bed. Mrs. Blackmore was an elderly lady admitted for a deep vein thrombosis. She also had diabetes, congestive heart failure, hypertension, asthma, atrial fibrillation, and S/P CVA with right hemiparesis. She had had two MI's in the past.

Dr. Perkins greeted Mrs. Blackmore and told her she wanted to listen to her lungs. She listened posteriorly, working her way inferiorly. Then she percussed her chest, but she said she did not hear increasing tone or dullness of sound. "She is not wheezing," Dr. Perkins reported.

Dr. Perkins moved her stethoscope anteriorly, again not hearing any abnormalities. She listened to the heart, starting at the base listening for aortic and pulmonic sounds. Then she moved down the sternal border to the apex and laterally to the axilla. Finally, she turned to Jonathan and said, "What did you hear?"

Jonathan replied, "Systolic murmur."

"What kind?" asked Dr. Perkins.

Jonathan leaned over the patient's bed again and listened to her chest. Then he said, "Holosystolic murmur, heard best at the lower sternal border."

"And?" said Perkins.

"Radiates to the axilla and, therefore, is a murmur of mitral regurgitation," finished Jonathan.

Perkins asked, "What else?" Then she herself listened again, over the sternal border and aortic areas. "What is that?" she asked the group.

They all answered, "Aortic sclerosis or aortic stenosis."

Dr. Perkins asked, "What's the difference?"

Jonathan answered, "Sclerosis is caused by atherosclerotic vessel disease. Stenosis is caused by stenotic valve."

Dr. Perkins continued her questioning. "How do you grade a murmur?"

Tom answered, "Grade 1 is barely audible."

Dr. Perkins murmured, "Usually heard only by staff. Grade 2?"

The students quickly supplied the following facts as in a ritual. "Audible with stethoscope. Grade 3—loudly with stethoscope. Grade 4—thrill, palpable murmur. Grade 5—a thrill with stethoscope slightly off the chest. Grade 6—can be heard with the stethoscope just over the chest, but not touching. From the door of the ward!" James sang out, finishing up the students' recital for that lesson on heart sounds.

Dr. Perkins bent down to the patient again to palpate the liver.

Coordinating Teaching Efforts

As this chapter has shown, the bedside is a remarkably rich setting for teaching medicine. To tap this instructional resource optimally, the attending physician and the resident need to coordinate their teaching efforts so they complement each other. The teaching done by the resident outside of attending rounds can prepare team members for attending rounds and can build upon the bedside teaching provided by the attending physician during rounds. This sort of team effort provides the structure, consistency, and reinforcement necessary to ensure maximal learning.

CHAPTER SIX

Providing Feedback

Anxious about the impact of the information on the trainee, but committed nonetheless to the need for feedback, the well-intentioned teacher talks around the problem or uses such indirect statements as to obfuscate the message entirely. The student, fearing a negative evaluation, supports and reinforces the teacher's avoidance. The result is that, despite the best of intentions, nothing of any real value gets transmitted or received. Even worse, concerns about the impact of feedback may lead to no feedback at all. (Ende, 1983)

The Attending Physician's Responsibility to Provide Feedback

Providing feedback is one of a teacher's most important responsibilities. Learners often need accurate descriptions of their errors and recommendations for improvement to correct inadequate performances. They also benefit from positive reinforcement when they are performing adequately or quite well. However, the intimidating prospect of delivering feedback and the daily rush of events frequently cause teachers to neglect opportunities for giving feedback. This phenomenon holds true across many educational settings and is well documented in clinical medical education (Bucher and Stelling, 1977; Weinholtz, 1981; Ways and Engel, 1982; Medio et al., 1984).

We recommend that attending physicians optimize their instruction by

1. looking for daily opportunities to offer feedback to individual team members and

2. scheduling midrotation conferences with individual team members to provide feedback on overall performance.

To implement these recommendations, it is valuable to adhere to some commonly accepted guidelines for giving feedback. While emphasizing that feedback is "an informed, nonevaluative, objective appraisal of performance intended to improve clinical skills—rather than an estimate of a trainee's personal worth," Ende (1983) offered such a set of guidelines. He indicated that feedback should be

- undertaken with the teacher and the trainee working as allies and with common goals;

- well timed and expected;

- based on firsthand data;

- regulated in quantity and limited to remediable behavior;

- phrased in descriptive, nonevaluative language;

- focused on specific performances, not generalizations;

- structured to include subjective data, as long as it is clearly labeled as such; and

- concerned with decisions and actions, rather than assumed intentions or interpretations.

Offering Daily Feedback

By alerting team members early in the rotation that regular feedback will be provided, attending physicians can prepare team members for the feedback process (Pratt and Magill, 1983; Linzer, 1984). Since feedback should be based on observed, firsthand data, it is unlikely that attendings can give every team member useful feedback every day, but each day some team members should be candidates for feedback. As Ende (1983) stated: "Any important part of the trainee's overall job is worthy of . . . feedback. A case presentation, the performance of a history and physical examination, a progress note, or observations made about a trainee's ability to conduct work rounds are all very appropriate."

Two incidents involving a physician particularly adept at providing timely feedback illustrate Ende's point regarding the abundance of opportunities for feedback.[1]

1. Weinholtz (1981) observed these incidents while conducting a participant-observation study. They have not been previously reported.

Frank, a third year student, gave a brief presentation to the team on boils (hidradenitis suppurative). While talking, he got up, went to the chalkboard, and made several drawings showing a boil during its stages of development.

After the presentation, Dr. Goff turned to the other team members and said, "Well, we're going to have to give Frank a grade on his presentation. Was that a good presentation? Could you repeat most of that presentation for us?"

Justine, another student responded, "I think so."

Goff asked "Why?"

Justine commented, "Well, it was pretty clear."

Goff continued, "But do you know what made it clear? It was the use of drawings. It is important to draw. . . . We can probably aid retention up to 35 percent with a good simple drawing. . . . Frank deserves an "A" for the clarity of his presentation. Now don't forget—use drawings in your presentations; when possible, even include them in your write-ups."

On a different occasion, Chris, another third year student, was presenting a patient who had been vomiting regularly for several days. While going over the results of his physical exam, Chris admitted that he had experienced difficulty hearing the patient's heart.

Dr. Goff asked, "Did you exercise him and have him lie on his left side? Did you have him do sit-ups and then listen while he was lying on his left side?"

"No, I didn't," Chris responded.

Dr. Goff then explained that these steps should be done whenever heart sounds are difficult to hear. She added that Chris should be careful to include them in the future.

Dr. Goff managed to use these two incidents not only to give feedback to particular individuals but also to make general points for all of the other team members. In the first case, this was not especially difficult to do because the feedback was positive. The second situation was more delicate because Chris had to be corrected in front of his peers. However, by focusing on Chris's behavior rather than on his merit as an individual, Goff was able to address Chris's learning need and make her point to the team without berating him.

Scheduling Conferences to Provide Feedback

Dr. Jeffries took me into his office, sat me down, asked me if I thought everything was going well, and gave me some midstream feedback. He offered a couple of ideas about things that he would like me to talk about during rounds. He told me how he thought everyone was performing. He even gave me some suggestions about my notes.

Even though an attending physician may provide daily feedback on specific incidents to particular individuals, students and house staff may not have a clear picture of their overall performance. If such a picture is not provided until they receive their final evaluations, there is no opportunity to improve performance during the rotation. Thus, it is wise to schedule a midrotation conference with each team member to provide an overall assessment of performance to that point.

In spite of the clear pedagogic benefits of such conferences, they are too rarely held. In one study, guidelines provided to attending physicians by the clerkship director specifically recommended midpoint feedback sessions. However, five of six attending physicians neglected to hold the sessions, and the one attending who held midrotation conferences did so with house staff only (Weinholtz, 1981). Commenting on a physician he had previously encountered who offered such feedback to students, one resident in this study remarked: "Dr. Michaels did that last year in pediatrics. He did it for all three students, which is really kind of a rarity. I think that it might be kind of a good idea, especially if they are not doing well. One girl hadn't been doing very good, and she seemed to perk up and do well the rest of the month. The other two had been doing fine. He just talked to them and let them know that they were doing a pretty good job. I think that is helpful too. It improves their spirits."

Before providing feedback, it is good practice to ask team members to assess their own performances. Self-assessment is a valuable skill that should be practiced throughout a health professional's education and career (Fuhrman and Weissburg, 1978). By asking a team member to assess his or her performance, the attending physician collects two valuable kinds of information. First, the attending finds out the weaknesses of which the team member is already aware. By allowing the student, intern, or resident to raise these concerns, the attending can avoid the awkwardness of having to raise a particular problem; the team member takes care of that. The attending can then adopt the positive stance of providing helpful suggestions regarding ways of confronting the problem. Second, the attending finds out the problem areas of which the individual is unaware or which the individual is hesitant to discuss. After dealing with the concerns that the team member previously raised, the attending can tactfully address these other issues, which may well involve matters such as interpersonal skills or professional attitudes.

Two references providing useful information on how to give and not give feedback are Schwenk and Whitman (1987) and Douglas et al. (1988). Their recommendations concerning feedback specificity, timeliness, clarity, and appropriateness fit well with those by Gordon (1978), who provided helpful suggestions for confronting and helping trainees who are demonstrating so-called attitude problems. Early identification and feedback play a critical role in the counseling approach Gordon recommended. He identified five steps in this counseling approach.

1. *Stating objectives:* Prior to any significant clinical rotation, students are oriented to the objectives for the rotation.

2. *Screening for potential problems:* During the rotation, data are collected on all major aspects of student performance. Exemplary performance is noted and reinforced, while problem performance is noted for corrective action. Such action may be handled through immediate feedback or through a conference when chronic problems arise. Clinical instructors must constantly keep the course objectives and level of student in mind when collecting data. Failure to do so may result in expecting either too much or too little of students.

3. *Clarifying problems:* If a chronic problem is detected, the instructor confronts the student in a private conference, interprets the problem, and opens the door for joint exploration of the root cause.

4. *Assessing specific behaviors:* To the extent that there is any disagreement between the instructor and the student over the nature of the problem, the student's specific performance record is analyzed. This step involves further clarification and will most likely be necessary only in situations where clear value differences exist.

5. *Providing assistance:* The instructor and student develop a plan to overcome whatever deficiency the student is experiencing. Such a plan may involve additional study (reading and so on), increased practice of certain skills, or attempts to interact with patients in a different manner.

If these steps do not lead to resolution of the identified problem, then extraordinary steps, including repeating the rotation, may be required. If this appears necessary, the attending physician's documentation of his or her efforts to help the student will aid the department in supporting the attending physician's recommendation that the student repeat.

Gordon's approach is consistent with our recommendation for midrotation feedback conferences. These sessions and other feedback opportunities can be facilitated by the attending's request for input regarding the quality of his or her teaching. Since team members may be reluctant to speak frankly with those in authority (Weinholtz, 1981), vague questions such as "How's it been going?" may not provide the attending with much useful information. Consequently, more specific questions will likely be necessary, for example, "Does my questioning interrupt your thinking during your presentations?" or "Are there other things that you would like me to demonstrate at the bedside?" The benefits of such questions extend beyond the information provided the attending. By allowing feedback to flow in two directions, the attending physician can create an environment conducive to constructive recommendations. Rather than solely conveying the message "I am sitting in judgment of you," the attending who solicits feedback communicates the message "We both should make efforts to improve our performance."

The Resident's Responsibility to Provide Feedback

Because residents and students work together so many hours of the day and night, residents have a unique opportunity to provide feedback to students and to each other. In no other training situation are so many hours spent working in such close proximity, as co-workers and as supervisor-learner teams. Residents can watch students perform tasks that attendings do not see, and residents can create opportunities for students and lower-level residents to learn that attendings cannot because of their relatively brief teaching encounters. Ende's guidelines for giving feedback (listed under "The Attending Physician's Responsibility to Provide Feedback" at the beginning of this chapter) are comprehensive and well applied to clinical education. We urge residents to study these guidelines from time to time and try to use them in their daily work and teaching. Here we will comment on several of these guidelines and provide examples.

Well-Timed and Expected Feedback

Feedback should be given daily and as soon as possible when the opportunity occurs in a learning situation. For the reasons mentioned above, residents are the first-line providers of feedback for medical students and for lower-level residents. Waiting until the end of a rotation to give feedback of a general nature provides no learning help. As residents go about their daily patient care, they can be giving each other and students informative feedback. It may be wise for the resident, at the beginning of the rotation, to mention that he or she will be giving feedback routinely.

The information may be corrective, that is, information that corrects erroneous or inaccurate information or demonstrates the correct method of performing a clinical procedure. Another type of feedback is confirmatory; the resident can confirm another learner's information or diagnostic impression. A third type of feedback is positive feedback. All types of informative feedback are useful. Here is an example of a resident giving a student positive feedback.

> Dr. Daniels, a first year medicine resident, was reviewing the case of Mrs. Williams, a 76-year-old woman with deep vein thrombosis, on work rounds. He said, "I have to commend John for taking the initiative to measure her legs. You can eyeball something and say, 'This leg is bigger than the other one,' but you can decide more precisely if you measure. John measured her legs on his own. He found that the right calf was larger than the left one."

Positive feedback is very satisfying to learners. As Ende pointed out, feedback of any type in medical training is scarce, but positive feedback is actually a rarity. John, the third year student who received this feedback, found it rewarding. He pursued other desirable but unrequired tasks throughout the rotation. This is also an example of specific feedback. Dr. Daniels mentioned John's specific action, measuring the patient's legs; he did not make a general statement.

Feedback Based on First-Hand Data

Feedback is best when it is based on first-hand observation (Ende, 1983). That is why residents are in the position of being the best providers of feedback. When feedback is given second- or third-hand, it often lacks specific detail and authenticity. Consider, for example, an attending physician telling a student at evaluation time, "Your resident says you don't do thorough physical exams." That feedback could have been more specific and would have had greater learning value if the resident, instead of the attending, had given it to the student when he or she observed the student doing the physical exam. Feedback can be based on partial first-hand observations. If the press of patient care does not allow a resident to observe an entire physical exam, he or she certainly can give feedback on the part of the exam observed. This partial feedback is much better than no feedback at all.

Feedback Focused on Specific Performance, Not Generalizations

General feedback is of little help to guide learning. Specific feedback, on the other hand, can help to change learning behavior.

Dr. Walberg, a second year medicine resident, was questioning Betty, a third-year student, about Mrs. Servicio's theophylline. Betty didn't know the information Dr. Walberg was asking. Dr. Walberg commented sharply, "You are treating your patient and you don't know what the normal dosage is. That's not good." Dr. Huntington, an intern, intervened on Betty's behalf. Walberg turned to Huntington and said, "I am instructing Betty; let's give her a chance to answer." Then he turned back to Betty and continued questioning her. Dr. Walberg concluded this interchange by saying directly to Betty, "You need to look up drug dosages. That is something we all must do whenever we encounter a drug with which we are unfamiliar. It is a good habit to have, and it is very important in providing excellent medical care." After the students left to go to their lecture, Walberg said to Huntington, "When I ask a student, don't answer for her. They (students) have to work and learn." Huntington agreed and took this correction affably.

Dr. Walberg gave specific feedback to a student and a resident in this instance. The specific feedback to the student was to learn normal drug dosages of medicine being used with patients for whom the student was responsible. The specific feedback to the intern was to stay out of the way when he, the resident in charge of the team, was instructing a student.

The two examples of feedback cited here illustrate two additional guidelines given by Ende. The residents in both examples, Dr. Daniels and Dr. Walberg, gave feedback that was concerned with decisions and actions rather than with assumed intentions or interpretations. Dr. Daniels commended a positive action the student had taken, measuring the patient's legs. Dr. Walberg pointed out to a student an action she should take—learning the dosages of medicines prescribed for her patient. Both examples of feedback are regulated in quantity and limited to remediable behavior.

In conclusion, residents can correct and reinforce learning by giving feedback frequently throughout the long hours they spend working with each other and students. Indeed, residents are the only teachers who are able to perform this valuable teaching function daily.

Some Final Comments

Clinical settings offer remarkable opportunities for both attending physicians and residents to give and to receive feedback. Taking advantage of these opportunities requires interpersonal skills that come more naturally to some individuals than to others. However, no matter what one's initial skill level, it is virtually always possible to refine or improve feedback behaviors. Developing this aspect of one's teaching repertoire deserves high priority among efforts to improve teaching. Results can be dramatic, with benefits spreading to many other interactions between teachers and learners.

CHAPTER SEVEN

Involving Other Health Professionals

Effective role modeling by physician faculty members skilled and comfortable in relating to other health professionals is essential if medical students are to receive adequate training in this important area. . . . Appropriate role modeling of teamwork skills should be an everyday departmental priority, and corrections should be made where problems are identified. (Geyman and Deyrup, 1984)

The Attending Physician and Other Health Professionals

The above recommendation by the Teamwork Skills Subgroup of the Project Panel on the General Professional Education of the Physician (GPEP) is particularly pertinent to teaching during attending rounds. A nationwide survey of internal medicine departments found that clinical pharmacists, nurses, physician assistants, social workers, and other health professionals were likely participants in attending rounds conducted in more than half of the reporting programs (Weinholtz et al., 1986b). The importance of such personnel was noted by Magraw (1966): "We physicians . . . are not actually able to deliver modern medical care by ourselves. . . . Most of these other professions now possess knowledge and skills which physicians, in any clinically usable way, do not have. We can be certain that an increasing number of such "paramedical" experts possessed of increasingly specialized skills will play an evermore important part in medical care teamwork."

Despite the presence of other health professionals during rounds and their obvious role in patient care, these individuals often slip into passive, secondary roles during rounds. The fact that attending rounds remain the preserve of physicians is illustrated by the lack of references to other health professions within the literature on attending rounds. Also, the sources likely to address interdisciplinary education during rounds do so tangentially, if at all (Ford, 1978; McGuire et al., 1983; Wylie, 1988). As Boufford (1978) commented, "interdisciplinary education occurs largely by chance in clinical settings where the needs of the patient or the situation compel traditionally oriented professionals to work together."

There are a few simple steps that attending physicians can take to increase the involvement of other health professionals during attending rounds and improve the team's interdisciplinary education. The attending can

1. regularly solicit participation in case discussions by nurses, social workers, or allied health professionals present during rounds and

2. occasionally request prepared presentations from these health professionals on content areas particularly suited both to their expertise and to problems encountered on the service.[1]

Soliciting Participation in Case Discussions

The attending physician can exert leadership by regularly inviting nonphysician health professionals to participate in patient case discussions.[2] By doing so, the attending can help overcome norms of passivity and deference which might prevent the team from freely engaging in disagreements potentially beneficial to patient care. Prescott and Bowen (1985) reported several types of such disagreements that might be dealt with efficiently during attending rounds rather than waiting for conflicts to arise after physicians make decisions without nurses input. The disagreements fell into three categories: general plan of care, specific orders, and patient disposition. Those focusing on general plan of care concerned the "extent or invasiveness of treat-

1. Weinholtz (1981) observed these two strategies practiced to a modest extent by a few attending physicians while conducting a participant-observation study; however, descriptions of the stategies were not included in the study's final report.

2. The attending physician might consider inviting one or two other health professionals to participate in attending rounds if they are not already doing so. For example, the head nurse on the service might be invited to join a group that has previously consisted solely of physicians and medical students.

ment, when to stop treating, and when not to resuscitate in the event of cardiac or respiratory arrest." Disagreements over specific orders dealt with "orders that nurses perceived as not in the patient's best interests, orders that conflicted with another order, or orders that asked a nurse to violate a policy." The final group of disagreements, those over patient disposition, "involved disputes regarding movement of patients from one unit to another and the timing of discharges."

For example, a disagreement addressing both the general plan of care and specific orders that could have been addressed during attending rounds was recounted by a staff nurse.

> Treating a patient in sickle cell crisis is an example of a disagreement between physicians and nurses that gets resolved by "sitting down and ironing it out." The patient is crying all the time saying, "I hurt so much," and the doctor is saying, "She can't have any more pain medication," and the nurse is saying, "We have to do something. We can't let her be in so much pain." So we went back and forth and the nurse would pull a few articles and say, "Why don't we put her on a morphine drip and that way she'll get less narcotic at a regular rate and she gets no exceptions?" And then one of the house staff came back and said, "Well let's just give her a placebo and see what happens there." And a lot of things have been tried, and it turned out that the morphine drip has been the best therapy for this girl. (Prescott and Bowen, 1985)

By skillfully soliciting the nurse's perspective on this case, the attending physician might have imbued attending rounds with a rich team perspective that is often missing. In doing so, the attending could have exhibited the type of teamwork skills that the GPEP Panel urged.

Another opportunity for interdisciplinary education is provided when discussing diabetes, an excellent example of a disease well suited for coordinated management and instructional efforts. By inviting a dietitian to attending rounds (if one is not already present), the attending physician can include in management discussions dietary instruction on controlling blood glucose. These discussions can also alert medical students and house staff to the dietitian's important role in diabetes management and education programs. The dietitian will probably bring an expertise that neither the attending physician nor the house staff and students possess. For example, even if these physicians and students are knowledgeable concerning food exchange lists and meal plans, they may not be aware of the effects of sick days, exercise, delayed meals, and alcohol on the insulin-dependent individual (Franz, 1981).

Requesting Prepared Presentations

Occasionally, the attending physician might want to go beyond including the nurse or allied health professional in management discussions and request a brief prepared presentation on a topic from the individual's area of expertise. Such talks can serve the same function as the brief presentations given by the attending physician (see Chapter 4) and are best requested when they are pertinent to the condition of a patient encountered on the service.

Clinical pharmacists are one example of allied health professionals who might be capable of delivering brief talks of instructional value to the entire team. The American Society of Hospital Pharmacists (1980) identified various topics upon which clinical pharmacists can provide useful information for health care teams. Attending rounds offer an ideal setting for clinical pharmacists to deliver presentations on topics such as new drugs, drug side effects and therapeutic risks, contraindications to particular drug therapies, and drug interactions (including drug-drug and drug-food interactions and laboratory test modifications).

Presentations on topics such as these need not take very long. Five to ten minutes of rounding time may be all that is necessary, and a few presentations per month are likely to suffice. Health professionals other than clinical pharmacists may also be asked to give occasional talks. For example, nurses and social workers might present on pertinent psychosocial and developmental issues or might explain the merits of particular patient education techniques. Again, dietitians may also make valuable contributions on a wide range of topics.

The Resident and Other Health Professionals

The residency training period is an excellent time for residents to learn teamwork with other health care professionals. Because they are still in training, residents tend to be somewhat more malleable during this period than later in their careers. Also, they do, in fact, have much to learn from other professionals.

To increase interdisciplinary education, we recommend that residents

1. establish a collegial atmosphere among the ward team and
2. actively solicit participation from other health care professionals.

Establishing a Collegial Atmosphere among the Ward Team

Residents, interns, pharmacy interns, dental residents, and students all are assigned to a ward team under the supervision of a senior resident. All share work responsibility and the condition of being learners. Social workers and nurses periodically interact with various members of the team. If the resident leader of the team sets a tone of cooperation and respect for the contribution of each member, then the other medical residents and students will tend to behave accordingly. Here is a negative example: a medical student who disparages the role of nurses in a patient's care. Residents can counteract this type of behavior and act positively.

> Tom, a fourth year student, was showing a patient chart to a new student on the first day of his third year. Tom flipped through a number of pages of the chart and said to his companion, "These are all nurses' notes. Don't pay any attention to that stuff. It's garbage. Just go directly to the real stuff—what the resident writes and the attending signs."

A resident who was standing nearby could have interjected that nurses can record important facts or perceptions about the patient and that their part in providing care to the patient should be acknowledged. Without collegiality and respect among the various care providers, the patient will suffer. Residents need to establish a positive tone for interdisciplinary education.

Actively Soliciting Participation from Other Health Care Professionals

Just as attending physicians can solicit participation on rounds from other health care professionals, residents can solicit

information and questions from pharmacy and dental interns
rotating on their team and from social workers and nurses. Here
is an example of an interdisciplinary team interacting on sit-
down rounds.

> Noreen, a second year medicine resident, listened to a student's up-
> date of his patient one morning in June. The team was seated in a
> small conference room usually reserved for families of patients on
> the general medicine ward. When the student finished his routine
> remarks, Noreen turned to Catherine, a pharmacy resident sitting
> on her left, and said, "What drugs are likely to induce fever?"
>
> Catherine replied lightly, "Almost any drug can cause fever." She
> flipped open her clinical manual of pharmacology and leafed
> through several pages and then said again, "Lots of drugs can cause
> fever."
>
> Noreen nodded and said, "Yes, that's true."

Although Catherine's answer wasn't very informative, both
the resident and the pharmacy intern obviously felt comfortable
with each other. The resident could have probed for more specific information or asked Catherine to present a brief summary
of drug-induced fever the following day. Further events demonstrated Catherine's value to the team.

> A little later during rounds, one of the students asked Catherine,
> "Should I give vitamin C for urinary infection?" Catherine quickly
> replied, "No."
>
> During the discussion of the last patient, some question arose
> about George's creatinine. Brenda, George's student doctor, asked
> Catherine if she would check the lab results with her. Catherine
> said, "Sure." Then they all laughed together spontaneously.
>
> As the team broke up, Noreen remarked to the research observer,
> "I think it's great to have Catherine on the team. She contributes.
> She's pretty quiet, but she looks up stuff for the team."

If a climate of collegiality has been established, all members
of the team will volunteer information freely and also ask questions whenever they need to obtain information. The informal
give and take of questioning and answering on work rounds, sit-
down rounds, and everywhere team members go is important to
learning.

Taking Teamwork Seriously

Erde (1982) suggested that modern health care teams are plagued by logical confusions and moral dilemmas. He argued that the "team" concept is typically used to imply a greater degree of coordination, understanding, commitment, and acceptance of health professional roles than actually exists and that team membership is used to promote solidarity against outside threats by establishing norms against whistleblowing.

In the complicated modern health care system, effective teamwork is essential to providing efficient, comprehensive care, but good teamwork requires conscious effort. As Lowe and Hirranen (1982) noted, teamwork is an evolutionary process that can occur only in a supportive environment emphasizing understanding, reflection, and practice. Inpatient rounds provide one setting where progress can be made on each of these fronts. Attending physicians and residents should lead the way.

CHAPTER EIGHT

Finishing the Rotation

As a rotation moves toward its conclusion, team members naturally begin thinking ahead to their next assignments and, as in any time-limited work group, an identifiable stage of group termination begins (Hare, 1976). This situation contains inherent educational pitfalls. As part of their normal withdrawal, team members are likely to look for areas where they can relax the fulfillment of their responsibilities. Since patient care cannot be slighted, educational responsibilities are a prime candidate for neglect.

Attending physicians and residents can accommodate this terminal phase of group development while still ensuring that important educational goals are met. Doing so requires some insight into group dynamics and some persistence.

The Attending Physician's Strategies

Although attending physicians might teach in many different ways during the rotation's closing phase, two strategies strike us as especially pertinent.

1. Adopt a less active role during rounds to foster team development and to better observe team members' interactions.

2. Conduct a private final evaluation conference with each team member.

Adopting a Less Active Role

Drawing on group development theory and qualitative research observations, Mattern et al. (1983) recommended that attending physicians initially adopt a directive teaching approach and progressively assume a more consultative posture as the rotation develops. No experimental studies have rigorously tested this recommendation, but a strong theoretical rationale supports such an approach.

Situational leadership theory (Hersey and Blanchard, 1988) posits four distinct styles of leadership available to attending physicians and other group leaders. The different approaches are determined by the amount of emphasis an attending physician places on task and relationship behaviors. "Task behaviors" focus directly on the type of work that is to be accomplished. "Relationship behaviors" focus on group processes and followers' interpersonal needs. The four categories defined by these two possibilities are (1) high task/low relationship ("telling"), (2) high task/high relationship ("selling"), (3) low task/high relationship ("participating"), and (4) low task/low relationship ("delegating"). Each of these four styles is illustrated in Table 4.

Along with Reddin (1967), Hersey and Blanchard proposed

Table 4. Styles of Situational Leadership Available to Attending Physicians

Style	Behavior of the Attending Physician
Telling (High task/low relationship)	Attending dominates communication by providing learners with information and/or directions concerning responsibilities expected of them in the future
Selling (High task/high relationship)	Attending closely controls the flow of communication but fosters two-way communication with learners and gives reinforcement for their contributions.
Participating (Low task/high relationship)	Attending stimulates free communication among the learners, offering occasional information and reinforcement as needed.
Delegating (Low task/low relationship)	Attending allows the learners to control the learning setting and serves primarily as an observer or low-profile participant.

Source: Adapted from Hersey, P., and Blanchard, K., (1988) *Management of organizational behavior* (5th ed.). Englewood Cliffs, N.J.: Prentice Hall, 171.

that each of these leadership styles may be more appropriate in certain situations and that a leader's effectiveness is determined by whether or not the leader can offer the appropriate leadership style when the situation demands it. Unlike Fiedler (1964), Hersey and Blanchard asserted that a leader can grow beyond dependence on a single dominant leadership style to develop a repertoire of styles. Thus, if trained to diagnose the leadership needs of the situation, an attending physician can adjust his or her behavior to enhance leadership effectiveness.

Hersey and Blanchard argued that, to make such adjustments, leaders should be able to diagnose individual and group "readiness." They defined readiness as "the extent to which a follower has the ability and willingness to accomplish a specific task." They defined ability as "the knowledge, experience, and skill that an individual or group brings to a particular task or activity" and willingness as "the extent to which an individual or group has the confidence, commitment and motivation to accomplish a specific task" (Hersey and Blanchard, 1988, p 174–175).

Situation leadership theory describes four readiness levels. The individual or group is (1) unable to perform a task and unwilling or insecure about attempting to perform it; (2) unable to perform a task but willing or confident (hence, inappropriately overconfident) about performing it; (3) able to perform a task but unwilling or insecure about doing so; or (4) able to perform a task and willing or confident about doing so. The art of leadership involves matching leadership styles to readiness levels in the manner indicated in Table 5. This typically involves a distinct progression toward delegation, but occasional "regressive cycles" to more directive approaches may be necessary when groups encounter responsibilities beyond their readiness levels (Hersey and Blanchard, 1988). For example, this might occur when the house staff and students are confronted by a case with which they have no prior experience and rapid decisions are necessary.

Notice that matching Readiness Level 1 with "Telling" corresponds closely to the type of "Orienting" that we described in Chapter 2. Similarly, the use of "Selling" and "Participating" correspond to most of the attending's teaching during the rotation, whether in the conference room or at the bedside. "Dele-

Table 5. The Progression of Levels of Group Readiness and Leadership Styles

Level of Group Readiness	Leadership Style
1. Low (unable and unwilling or insecure)	Telling
2. Low-moderate (unable but willing or confident)	Selling
3. Moderate-high (able but unwilling or insecure)	Participating
4. High (able/competent and willing/confident	Delegating

Source: Adapted from Hersey, P., and Blanchard, K. (1988) *Management of organizational behavior* (5th ed.). Englewood Cliffs, N.J.: Prentice Hall, 180.

gating," however, calls for the attending physician to move his or her instruction to a new level. It requires recognizing that the team has developed sufficiently to function with little or no overt direction by the attending. It demands breaking the dependence that group leaders so often foster out of ignorance or their own insecurity.

Moving to the "Delegating" style during the last week of a rotation offers distinct educational advantages. Foremost, by adopting an observer stance, the attending physician can obtain a different perception of team members' abilities than that obtained when the attending is at the center of all the action. In the latter circumstance, it is often difficult to distinguish the attending's own influence on the situation.

During case discussions, will the team pick up on psychosocial issues without the attending's prompting them? Several observations might tell and also provide the attending with new opportunities for offering feedback. How much of a student's difficulty presenting a case is due to the student's limitations, and how much is due to the attending's intimidating questioning? To gauge this, the attending might allow other team members to play the attending's role during the student's case presentations, while the attending observes the process. This strategy not only achieves the desired effect of minimizing the attending's influence but also allows the team member hearing the case the opportunity to become involved in a more active manner. By actively experiencing the dilemma of receiving either too little or too much information, the team member serving as an attending might well gain insights for improving his or her own presentations (Weinholtz, 1983b). The benefits of this approach are explained by the following quotation from an attending physician who uses it.

> It's one way to pull everybody into the case. During presentations, it is very easy for the other members of the team to fall asleep. My use of this strategy stems from my own personal experience. On my first day as a fellow, my attending on the consult service asked a student to present to me. It just rocked me in my boots, but it was a very good experience. It is especially good when there are only one or two patients that have to be presented, so you can spend the time that is needed. The only thing that you have to be careful of is turning the role of the attending over to someone who is not ready for it.

The attending's caution might be expanded even more. The traditions and norms of attending rounds are so ingrained and revolve so much around the attending physician as the central figure that any effort by the attending to adopt a lower profile is likely to confuse team members. Therefore, the shift should be gradual but also explicit. Obviously, the attending can never completely withdraw from the team, as his or her input is often legally required. However, the attending can gently but clearly alert the team that on occasion he or she will prefer to watch to see how the team handles things on its own.

Conducting Final Evaluation Conferences

Too often, team members receive written final evaluations from their rotations without the benefit of a face-to-face explanation by their attending physicians. As indicated by these two students' comments, such evaluation forms frequently provide insufficient information and may well contain unpleasant surprises.

> My last attending was a real easygoing guy. He didn't tell you what he didn't like about you, so there was no way to try to improve. When I got my evaluations, he gave me a "satisfactory," but he wrote down a whole bunch of stuff that he'd never told me about. (Student 1)

The evaluations that they give you are just totally inadequate. . . . I just got back an evaluation form six months after I was down in Wilmington. My attending didn't even do it, and the guy who filled it out didn't write any comments at all. He just took a pen and made a big circle around all of the 3s.

Another attending of mine just wrote, "Bart will make a fine physician." I mean, he could have written more than that. It would have only taken five minutes. After all, they expect us to write careful evaluations of the clerkship. You think that they would be willing to do the same for us. (Student 2)

The problem is not experienced by students alone. Nor, as this resident's comments indicate, is it simply the fault of the more negligent attending physicians.

You know, I really liked working with Dr. Waitzman. It was just an exceptionally good experience . . . but I have to add a criticism. He never sat down with any of the house staff to tell them how he thought that they had performed. That sort of thing can be very helpful.

The logical culmination to the feedback provided by the attending physician throughout the rotation (see Chapter 6) is a private final evaluation conference at the rotation's close. While clinical evaluation of medical students and house staff poses recurring problems for which there is no single solution (Stemmler, 1986; Tonesk, 1986), frank final evaluation conferences with individual team members are a positive step that can substantially improve clinical evaluation efforts. Whether a team member performs excellently or has trouble focusing on what is important, demonstrates a limited knowledge base, is disorganized, is too casual, or is "all thumbs," it is important that he or she leave the rotation knowing the attending physician's final assessment of the skills exhibited. Along with this assessment should come recommendations for efforts to improve future performance.

The feedback that the attending offers during the rotation is absolutely critical to making such final conferences effective learning experiences. If the attending has offered sufficient feedback all along the way, the final conference should actually offer no great surprises. In fact, except in the rare cases of particularly recalcitrant team members, these sessions should offer final confirmation that team members have made progress on areas previously noted and specified for attention.

Clinical faculty often feel inadequately prepared to evaluate problem students and are hesitant to record negative evaluations (Tonesk and Buchanan, 1987). Reticence in these murky areas of negative evaluation is understandable but not condonable. Team members experiencing difficulty must be confronted and their performance problems documented, or clinical evaluation systems break down. One of the things that faculty need to know to give them the confidence to confront and document is that their "educated guesses" and "personal judgments" constitute legitimate evaluation data, especially when evaluating "personal and professional qualities and more complex cognitive and clinical skills" (Tonesk and Buchanan, 1987). However, such assessments carry weight only if they have been based on extended observations. Thus, attending physicians must be observant from the start of the rotation and promptly provide feedback on problem areas accompanied by specific suggestions for improvement. If these conditions are met, faculty can conduct final conferences and complete final evaluations with the conviction that they have appropriately fulfilled their responsibilities.

Dr. Jeffries's comments on how he handles his final evaluation conferences indicate one approach that might be taken and a rationale for doing so.

> I filled out the evaluation forms with the students, on a one-to-one basis. I had the evaluation form here. I read the qualification, and I asked each student to rank himself. After he did so, I ranked him. Then, if we differed, we discussed our reasons.
>
> I think that it is part of the learning process to evoke from the student his impressions of himself or his performance and to hear somebody else's impression. I think a student needs to know where he stands. He needs to know if he is doing an outstanding job in one area or needs some improvement in another area. The only way you can improve is if you know what your problems are.

A final point seems worth adding. Final evaluation conferences provide attending physicians with one last chance to solicit information on ways that they might adjust their teaching to meet individuals' specific needs. A question such as, "Is there any way I could have helped you more than I did?" can efficiently garner valuable information for improving teaching efforts.

The Resident's Strategies

Residents can be most helpful if they play a cooperative role with attendings toward the end of the rotation. They can cooperate by allowing students more independence of action and by being prepared to participate in evaluating the students.

Delegating Autonomy

In accord with the recommendation to attendings to delegate more autonomy to the team, residents can allow students a little more freedom or opportunity to take the initiative in patient care and in their own learning. Instead of routinely telling students, they can remain silent and watch to see if students do the necessary patient care tasks within their sphere of responsibility. Of course, if a student does not perform the task, the resident or intern must call it to the student's attention or perform the task.

Evaluating Team Members

The most prominent job at the end of a rotation is the evaluation of the team. To be prepared for evaluation at the end, residents should find out at the beginning of the rotation what responsibilities they will have for evaluating students and lower-level residents. Ideally, departments should have policies defining the evaluation role of residents at each level. If this role has not been defined, chief residents should work to formulate such a policy statement. However, individual residents must deal with situations in which their role is ambiguous. Therefore, we say to individual residents that they must take the initiative to find out from the attending physician at the beginning of the rotation what role they will be expected to play in evaluating other learners on the team.

In general, residents should try to evaluate the attainment of the objectives. The amount of scutwork done is secondary to (or incidental to) learning. Personal likes or differences should not color the subjective judgment of the performance of learning tasks. Despite the thinking of some attending physicians, residents are very capable of evaluating the degree of skill in taking histories and performing physical exams and simple procedures such as phlebotomy, venipuncture, and the like. In fact, because residents spend so much time with students, they usually have had more opportunity to observe these tasks. Residents can be valuable assistants to attendings in the evaluation of students.

Sometimes the evaluation of the learner by the resident is only an opinion delivered orally to the attending. Even in this situation the best way to prepare an evaluation is to write brief notes periodically about the learners' performance. These notes should be jottings of critical incidents and comments about the quality of performance of assigned tasks. For example, one day the resident, Dr. Climes, noted that Stephen always saw each of his assigned patients before work rounds and that he was on time for work rounds. Another note was that he had observed Stephen take a very thorough history and physical of a new patient that night on call. A third note indicated that Stephen didn't take initiative to practice procedures, although two opportunities had occurred that day. Such notes give focus and detail to document a resident's impressions of a student's performance throughout the rotation.

The resident also can give some final oral feedback *directly to the student* about his or her performance. Some students, especially those who have put forth a good effort, really want such feedback. The resident's feedback can be reinforcing of attitudes and habits that physicians in training must acquire: assuming responsibility, being careful, and being prepared. A few minutes of private conversation with the resident can bring the rotation to conclusion with satisfaction for both resident and student.

Providing Effective Closure

The final week of a rotation offers valuable educational opportunities for all team members. It is important that attending physicians and residents recognize this and that they tailor their teaching efforts to take advantage of team members' predictable needs for autonomy and feedback. The transition to these final teaching behaviors should not be abrupt. Indeed, the rotation should steadily progress in their direction so the events of the final week are a logical culmination to all that has preceded.

CHAPTER NINE

The Continuing Challenge of Improving One's Teaching

Many writers, including me, say teaching is an art. What does it mean to speak of an "art" of teaching? Teaching is an instrumental or practical art, not a fine art aimed at creating beauty for its own sake. As an instrumental art, teaching is something that departs from recipes, formulas, or algorithms. It requires improvisation; spontaneity; the handling of hosts of considerations of form, style, pace, rhythm; and appropriateness. (Gage, 1985, p. 4)

As with improving any "art," improving teaching is an ongoing challenge. It requires reflecting on current teaching practices, searching for alternative approaches, experimenting with the appealing alternatives, and obtaining a desirable balance of the old and the new. For even the best teachers, this is a lifelong process. There are always refinements that can be considered and adjustments that can be made.

This book has presented many specific recommendations for improving teaching during rounds. We reiterate briefly.

Starting the Rotation

The Attending Physician

1. Clearly orient all team members to your expectations for the rotation.
2. Solicit information from all team members regarding their abilities, interests, and expectations for the rotation.
3. Establish a climate conducive to learning.

The Resident

1. State your expectations.
2. Solicit information from students and interns for planning instruction.
3. Establish a positive learning climate.

Allocating Time for Teaching
The Attending Physician

1. Personally review charts and visit patients before attending rounds to reserve a maximal amount of attending round time for teaching.
2. Conduct special teaching sessions for medical students.

The Resident

1. Be prepared to take advantage of "teachable moments" that occur throughout the day.
2. Plan activities for the succeeding day at the close of the current day. In the morning, review the day's activities and adjust plans if changes are necessary. Divide and assign the team's tasks to achieve maximal efficiency.

Teaching in the Conference Room
The Attending Physician

1. Limit interruptions of the case presentations by students and house staff, reserving the majority of questions and comments until after the presentations are completed.
2. After case presentations, actively engage in discussions, using probing questions to assess understanding and to provoke thought. Depending on the learner and the particular case, these questions may be used to assess the learner's ability to grasp factual knowledge, comprehend key concepts, apply basic principles, analyze complex situations, or evaluate courses of action.
3. Frequently use illustrative devices (e.g., chalkboard, x-ray viewer, EKG tape, etc.) to emphasize important information and make abstract points more concrete.

4. Deliver occasional, brief talks on pertinent topics from your subspecialty area or on general topics in which you are particularly well versed.

5. Provide team members with relevant readings or references and encourage team members to share information obtained through their readings and consultations.

The Resident

1. Make patient care a learning experience.

2. a. Simultaneously direct the work and learning.
   b. Use probing questions to provoke thought.
   c. Point out things to learn.

3. Use illustrations and diagrams.

4. Encourage and direct reading in conjunction with or as a supplement to the attending's assigned reading.

Teaching at the Bedside

The Attending Physician

1. Use the patient for effective teaching whenever possible.

2. Make bedside teaching explicit. When possible, alert team members beforehand to skills that will be demonstrated at the bedside. Whether or not forewarning is possible, address bedside interactions in follow-up discussions.

3. Focus on teaching both physical skills (e.g., conducting a physical exam) and interpersonal skills (e.g., eliciting an accurate history or addressing the patient's personal needs).

4. When possible, observe team members as they perform the physical and interpersonal skills that you have demonstrated and give them feedback on their performances.

5. Generally, reserve case presentations for the conference room; if requiring presentations at the bedside, however take precautions to avoid causing patients distress.

6. Be conscious of the time demands placed on team members. Make bedside visits concise. Rather than requiring all team members to visit all patients during rounds, consider having team members visit only their own patients and specific patients from whom they might learn a great deal.

7. Use the hallway efficiently. Limit the time spent on patient presentations and discussions in the hallway and minimize probing questions. If lengthy follow-up discussions are required, move to the conference room.

The Resident

During attending rounds:

1. Elaborate on what the attending is explaining or demonstrating.
2. Prompt students to give answers and responses.
3. Elicit teaching from the attending.

During work rounds and at other times of the day:

4. Reinforce or correct the attending's teaching.
5. Teach clinical procedures.
6. Teach history-taking and physical examination skills.

Providing Feedback

The Attending Physician

Using Ende's guidelines (listed below):

1. Look for daily opportunities to offer individual team members feedback.
2. Schedule midrotation and end of rotation conferences with individual team members to provide feedback on overall performance.

The Resident

Provide feedback (using Ende's guidelines):

1. Undertake feedback as an ally of the student, working toward common goals.
2. Give feedback that is well timed and expected.
3. Base feedback on firsthand data.
4. Regulate feedback in quantity and limit it to remediable behavior.
5. Phrase feedback in descriptive, nonevaluative language.
6. Focus on specific performances, not generalizations.
7. Include subjective data, but label it as such.

8. Be concerned with decisions and actions, not assumed intentions or interpretations.

Involving Other Health Professionals
The Attending Physician

1. Regularly solicit participation in case discussions by nurses, social workers, or allied health professionals present during rounds.
2. Occasionally request prepared presentations from these health professionals on content areas particularly suited both to their expertise and to problems encountered on the service.

The Resident

1. Establish a collegial atmosphere among the ward team.
2. Actively solicit participation from other health care professionals.

Finishing the Rotation
The Attending Physician

1. Adopt a less active role during rounds for better observation of team members' interactions.
2. Conduct a private final evaluation conference with each team member.

The Resident

Cooperate with the attendings' strategies toward the end of the rotation.

1. Allow students more independence of action.
2. Prepare to participate in evaluating the students.

In combination, the recommendations on this list constitute a daunting challenge for anyone interested in improving his or her teaching. However, simply by selecting one or two recommendations before a rotation, an attending physician or resident can experiment with a manageable number of new teaching behaviors. Gradually, over a year or two, one's teaching repertoire can be expanded substantially.

This sort of individual trial-and-error method, following

personal reading and reflection, might also be used to implement clinical teaching suggestions from other sources, such as Schwenk and Whitman (1987) or Douglas et al. (1988). It is a very legitimate way to improve teaching. Still, it is only one of many available techniques. In a fine literature review, Stritter (1983) examined a variety of other teaching improvement strategies, including

- being observed by an educational consultant and receiving feedback based on the observations,[1]

- participating in collaborative educational research projects,

- participating in teaching-oriented fellowships or degree programs,

- attending instructional workshops, and

- utilizing insights obtained from self-assessments, peer assessments, and student assessments based upon specific evaluative criteria.

One's ability to draw upon these strategies depends greatly on the extent to which one's department, medical school, and teaching hospital tangibly support efforts to improve teaching (Irby, 1986). If blessed with abundant support, various opportunities for personal development will surface throughout the year. If not, it will probably be necessary to develop one's own opportunities creatively.

Typically, every department contains several individuals for whom teaching is an especially high priority. These colleagues can be organized into a group that, much like a journal club, meets once a month to discuss instructional topics and share information concerning continuing medical education courses offered locally or elsewhere. Also, many medical schools now have small offices of educational research and development staffed by Ph.D.s in the behavioral sciences who are willing to work with individual faculty members or entire departments on efforts to improve teaching. Often, valuable collaborative projects can be established with these offices.

Turning elsewhere, the annual meeting of the Association of American Medical Colleges (AAMC) consistently provides a se-

---

1. Skeff (1983) and Weinholtz et al. (1989) developed approaches suitable for consultants to provide attending physicians with feedback. Edwards et al. (1988b) described a program for doing so with residents.

ries of high-quality workshops and symposia on instructional issues, as does the Annual Conference of the Generalists in Medical Education, which is held concurrent with the AAMC annual meeting. At these national gatherings, you can learn a great deal about teaching while establishing a network of colleagues around the nation who share similar educational interests.

Finally, among several faculty development programs that exist nationwide, Dr. Kelley Skeff has taken a unique step at Stanford University by establishing a faculty development program focusing specifically on helping clinicians improve their teaching. Designed to educate faculty members who can return to their institutions and train their colleagues, the Stanford program emphasizes clinical teaching theory and practice. Those instructed at Stanford participate in discussions, seminars, lectures, analysis of videotapes, and practice with feedback. The program includes extensive evaluation during and after the time at Stanford. By attracting faculty from institutions throughout the nation and abroad, Skeff is building a consortium capable of studying ways of improving clinical teaching at many different teaching hospitals.

Clearly, there are many possible routes to becoming a better teacher, but all require persistence and dedication to improvement. Whatever route you choose, we hope this book will be helpful to you along the way.

REFERENCES

Adams, W. R., Ham, T. H., Mawardi, B. H., Scali, H. A., and Weisman, R. A. (1964) A naturalistic study of teaching in a clinical clerkship. *Journal of Medical Education,* 39:164–166.

American Society of Hospital Pharmacists (1980) ASHP and ANA guidelines for collaboration of pharmacists and nurses in institutional care settings. *American Journal of Hospital Pharmacy,* 37: 253–254.

Anderson, J. R. (1985) *Cognitive psychology and its implications* (2nd ed.). New York: W.H. Freeman and Co.

Apter, A., Metzger, R., and Glassroth, J. (1988) Residents' perceptions of their role as teachers. *Journal of Medical Education,* 63:900–905.

Arluke, A. (1980) Roundsmanship: Inherent control on a medical teaching ward. *Social Science and Medicine,* 14a:297–302.

Asch, D. A., and Parker, R. M. (1988) The Libby Zion case. *New England Journal of Medicine,* 318(12):771–775.

Association of American Medical Colleges (1981) Graduate medical education: Proposals for the eighties. *Journal of Medical Education,* 56(9 part 2).

Association of American Medical Colleges (1984) Physicians for the twenty-first century. *Journal of Medical Education,* 59(11 part 2).

Becker, H., Geer, B., Hughes, E., and Strauss, A. (1961) *Boys in white.* Chicago: University of Chicago Press.

Boufford, J. I. (1978) Interdisciplinary clinical education. In C.W. Ford (ed.): *Clinical education for the allied health professions.* St. Louis: C.V. Mosby, 59–65.

Brownell, A.K.W., and McDougall, G. M. (1984) The patient as the focus of teaching. *Canadian Medical Association Journal,* 131: 855–857.

Bucher, R., and Stelling, J. G. (1977) *Becoming professional.* Beverly Hills, Calif.: Sage Publications.

117

Camp, M. G., Hoban, J. D., and Katz, P. A. (1985) Course on teaching for house officers. *Journal of Medical Education,* 60:140–142.

Coombs, R. (1978) *Mastering medicine.* New York: The Free Press.

Coppernoll, P. S., and Davies, D. F. (1974) Goal-oriented evaluation of teaching methods by medical students and faculty. *Journal of Medical Education,* 49:424–430.

Daggett, C. J. (1977) *A study to determine the role of attending physicians in the clinical training of medical students and resident physicians.* Unpublished doctoral dissertation. Amherst: University of Massachusetts.

Dawson, D. J., and Patel, V. L. (1983) Bedside encounter and clinical performance of junior clinical clerks. In *Proceedings of the Twenty-Second Annual Research in Medical Education Conference.* Washington, D.C.: Association of American Medical Colleges, 186–191.

Dick, W., and Carey, L. (1985) *The systematic design of instruction* (2nd ed.). Glenview, Ill.: Scott, Foresman and Co.

Douglas, K. C., Hosokawa, M. C., and Lawler, F. H. (1988) *A practical guide to clinical teaching in medicine.* New York: Springer.

Edwards, J. C. (1990) Using classic and contemporary visual images in clinical teaching. *Academic Medicine,* 65(5):297–298.

Edwards, J. C., and Marier, R. L. (1988) *Clinical teaching for medical residents.* New York: Springer.

Edwards, J. C., Kissling, G. E., Plauché, W. C., and Marier, R. L. (1986) Long-term evaluation of training residents in clinical teaching skills. *Journal of Medical Education,* 61:967–970.

Edwards, J. C., Kissling, G. E., Brannan, J. R., Plauché, W. C., and Marier, R. L. (1988a) Study of teaching residents how to teach. *Journal of Medical Education,* 63:603–609.

Edwards, J. C., Kissling, G. E., Plauché, W. C., and Marier, R. L. (1988b). Developing and evaluating a teaching improvement program for residents. In J. C. Edwards and R. L. Marier (eds.): *Clinical teaching for medical residents.* New York: Springer, 157–174.

Ende, J. (1983) Feedback in clinical medical education. *Journal of the American Medical Association,* 250:777–781.

Engel, G. L. (1971). The deficiencies of the case presentation as a method of clinical teaching. *New England Journal of Medicine,* 284(11):20–24.

Erde, E. L. (1982) Logical confusions and moral dilemmas in health care teams and team talk. In G. Agich (ed.): *Responsibility in health care.* Dordrecht, Holland: D. Reidel Publishing Co., 193–213.

Erickson, S. C. (1984) *The essence of good teaching.* San Francisco: Jossey-Bass Publishers.

Fiedler, F. E. (1964). *A theory of leadership effectiveness.* New York: McGraw-Hill.

Foley, R. P., and Smilansky, J. (1980) *Teaching techniques: A handbook for health professionals.* New York: McGraw-Hill.

Foley, R., Smilansky, J., and Yonke, A. (1979) Teacher-student interaction in a medical clerkship. *Journal of Medical Education,* 54:622–626.

Ford, C. W. (ed.) (1978) *Clinical education for the allied health professions.* St. Louis: C.V. Mosby.

Franz, M. (1981) The dietician: A key member of the diabetes team. *Journal of the American Dietetic Association,* 79:302–305.

Fuhrman, B. S., and Weissburg, M. J. (1978) Self-assessment. In M. K. Morgan and D. M. Irby (eds.): *Evaluating clinical competence in the health professions.* St. Louis: C. V. Mosby.

Gage, N. L. (1985) *Hard gains in the soft sciences: The case of pedagogy.* Bloomington, Ind.: Phi Delta Kappa.

Gagne, E. D. (1985) *The cognitive psychology of school learning.* Boston: Little, Brown.

Geyman, J. P., and Deyrup, J. A. (1984) Subgroup report on teamwork skills. Physicians for the twenty-first century: Report of the project panel of the general professional education of the physician and college preparation for medicine. *Journal of Medical Education,* 59(11):169–172.

Gordon, M. J. (1978) Assessment of student affect: A clinical approach. In M. K. Morgan and D. M. Irby (eds.): *Evaluating clinical competence in the health professions.* St. Louis: C. V. Mosby.

Gordon, T. (1977) *Leader effectiveness training.* New York: Wyden Books.

Hare, A. P. (1976) *Handbook of small group research* (2nd ed.). New York: The Free Press.

Harvard Medical School Office of Educational Development (1989) The new pathway to general medical education at Harvard University. *Teaching and Learning in Medicine,* 1:42–46.

Hersey, P., and Blanchard, K. (1988) *Management of organizational behavior* (5th ed.). Englewood Cliffs, N.J.: Prentice Hall.

Hinz, C. F. (1966) Direct observation as a means of teaching and evaluating clinical skills. *Journal of Medical Education,* 41:150–161.

Irby, D. (1978) Clinical teacher effectiveness in medicine. *Journal of Medical Education,* 53:808–815.

Irby, D. (1986) Clinical teaching and the clinical teacher. *Journal of Medical Education,* 61(9 part 2):35–45.

Jason, H. R. (1962) A study of medical teacher practices. *Journal of Medical Education,* 37:258–261.

Jewett, L. S., Greenberg, L. W., and Goldberg, R. M. (1982) Teaching residents how to teach: A one-year study. *Journal of Medical Education,* 57:361–366.

Kassirer, J. P. (1983) Iterative hypothesis testing: Let's preach what we practice. *New England Journal of Medicine,* 309:921–925.

Kaufman, A. (1989) Commentary on "Making doctors—a new approach." *Teaching and Learning in Medicine,* 1:67.

Kemp, K. (1985) *The instructional design process.* New York: Harper and Row.

Knowles, M. (1973) *The adult learner: A neglected species.* Houston: Gulf Publishing Co.

Lawson, B. K., and Harvill, L. M. (1980) The evaluation of a training program for improving residents' teaching skills. *Journal of Medical Education,* 55:1001–1005.

Linfors, E. W., and Neelon, F. A. (1980) The case for bedside rounds. *New England Journal of Medicine,* 303(21):1230–1233.

Linzer, M. (1984) Feedback in medical education. *Journal of the American Medical Association,* 251:277.

Lowe, J. I., and Herranen, M. (1982) Understanding teamwork: Another look at the concepts. *Social Work in Health Care,* 7(2):1–11.

Lurie, N., Rank, B., Parenti, C., Wooley, T., and Snoke, W. (1989) How do house officers spend their nights? *New England Journal of Medicine,* 320:1673–1677.

Magraw, R. M. (1966) *Ferment in medicine.* Philadelphia: W. B. Saunders.

Mangione, C. M. (1986) How medical school did and did not prepare me for graduate medical education. *Journal of Medical Education,* 61(9 part 2):3–10.

Mattern, W. D., Weinholtz, D., and Friedman, C. P. (1983) The attending physician as teacher. *New England Journal of Medicine,* 308:1129–1132.

Maxwell, J. A., Cohen, R. M., and Reinhard, J. D. (1983) A qualitative study of teaching rounds in a department of medicine. In *Proceedings of the Twenty-Second Annual Research in Medical Education Conference.* Washington, D.C.: Association of American Medical Colleges, 283–288.

McCall, T. B. (1989) No turning back: A blueprint for residency reform. *Journal of the American Medical Association,* 261(6):909–910.

McGuire, C. H., Foley, R. P., Gorr, A., Richards, R. W., and associates (1983) *Handbook of Health Professions Education.* San Francisco: Jossey-Bass Publishers.

Medio, F. J., Wilkerson, L., Maxwell, J. A., Cohen, R. M., and Reinhard, J. D. (1984) Improving teaching rounds: Action research in medical education. In *Proceedings of the Twenty-Third Annual Research in Medical Education Conference.* Washington, D.C.: Association of American Medical Colleges, 283–288.

Miller, S. J. (1968) *The educational experience of interns.* Waltham, Mass.: Brandeis University.

Mumford, E. (1970) *Interns: From students to physicians.* Cambridge, Mass.: Harvard University Press.

Osler, W. (1903) On the need of a radical reform in our methods of teaching senior students. *Med News,* 82:49–53.

Payson, H. E., and Barchas, J. D. (1965) A time study of medical teaching rounds. *New England Journal of Medicine,* 273:1468–1471.

Payson, H. E., Gaenslen, E. C., and Stargardter, F. L. (1961) Time study of an internship on a university medical service. *New England Journal of Medicine,* 264:439–443.

Petzel, R. A., Harris, I. B., and Masler, D. S. (1982) The empirical validation of clinical teaching strategies. *Evaluation and the Health Professions,* 5:499–508.

Plauché, W. C., and Edwards, J. C. (1988) Images and emotion in patient-centered clinical teaching. *Perspectives in Biology and Medicine,* 31(4):602–609.

Pratt, D., and Magill, M. K. (1983) Education contracts: A basis for effective clinical teaching. *Journal of Medical Education,* 58:462–467.

Prescott, P. A., and Bowen, S. A. (1985) Physician-nurse relationships. *Annals of Internal Medicine,* 103:127–133.

Reddin, W. J. (1967) The 3-D management style theory. *Training and Development Journal,* 21:8–17.

Reichsman, F., Browning, F. E., and Hinshaw, J. R. (1964) Observations of undergraduate clinical teaching in action. *Journal of Medical Education,* 39:147–153.

Romano, J. (1941) Patient's attitudes and behavior in ward round teaching. *Journal of the American Medical Association,* 117(9):664–667.

Russell, I. J. (1985) Condition diagramming: A new approach to teaching clinical integration. *Medical Education,* 19:220–225.

Schor, E. L., and Grayson, M. (1984) Outstanding clinical teachers: Methods, characteristics and behaviors. *Proceedings of the Twenty-Third Annual Research in Medical Education Conference.* Washington, D.C.: Association of American Medical Colleges, 271–276.

Schwenk, T. L., and Whitman, N. A. (1987) *The physician as teacher.* Baltimore: Williams & Wilkins.

Shankel, S. W., and Mazzaferri, E. L. (1986) Teaching the resident in internal medicine: Present practices and suggestions for the future. *Journal of the American Medical Association,* 256(6):725–729.

Sheehan, K. H., Sheehan, D. V., White, K., Leibowitz, A., and Baldwin, D.W.C. (1990) A pilot study of medical student abuse. *JAMA,* 263(4):533–537.

Siegel, B. (1986) *Love, Medicine and Miracles.* New York: Harper and Row.

Silver, H. K., and Glichen, A. D. (1990) Medical student abuse. *JAMA,* 263(4):527–531.

Skeff, K. M. (1983) Evaluation of a method for improving the teaching performance of the attending physician. *American Journal of Medicine,* 75:465–470.

Skeff, K. M., Campbell, M., Stratos, G., Jones, H. W., and Cooke, M. (1984) Assessment by attending physicians of a seminar method to improve clinical teaching. *Journal of Medical Education,* 59:944–950.

Skeff, K. M., Campbell, M., and Stratos, G. (1985) Process and product in clinical teaching: A correlation study. In *Proceedings of the Twenty-Fourth Annual Research in Medical Education Conference.* Washington, D.C.: Association of American Medical Colleges, 25–29.

Stemmler, E. J. (1986) Promoting improved evaluation of students during clinical education: A complex management task. *Journal of Medical Education,* 61(9, part 2):75–81.

Steward, D. E., and Feltovich, P. (1988) Why residents should teach: The parallel processes of teaching and learning. In J. C. Edwards and R. L. Marier (eds.): *Clinical teaching for medical residents: Roles, techniques, and programs.* New York: Springer.

Stritter, F. (1983) Faculty evaluation and development. In C. H. McGuire, R. P. Foley, A. Gorr, R. W. Richards, and associates (eds.): *Handbook of Health Professions Education.* San Francisco: Jossey-Bass, 294–318.

Stritter, F. T., and Flair, M. D. (1980) *Effective clinical teaching.* Bethesda, Md.: National Medical Audiovisual Center.

Stritter, F. T., Hain, J. D., and Grimes, D. A. (1975) Clinical teaching reexamined. *Journal of Medical Education,* 50:876–882.

Tiberius, R. G., Slingerland, J. M., Sachin, H. D., Jubas, K., Bell, M., and Matlow, A. (1987) The impact of student evaluative feedback on the improvement of clinical teaching. Paper presented at the annual meeting of the American Educational Research Association, Washington, D.C.

Tonesk, X. (1986) AAMC program to promote improved evaluation of students during clinical education. *Journal of Medical Education,* 61(9 part 2):83–88.

Tonesk, X., and Buchanan, R. G. (1987) An AAMC pilot study by 10 medical schools of clinical evaluation of students. *Journal of Medical Education,* 62(9):707–718.

Tremonti, L. P., and Biddle, W. B. (1982) Teaching behaviors of residents and faculty members. *Journal of Medical Education,* 57: 854–859.

Ways, P. O., and Engle, J. D. (1982) A sociocultural view of clerkship education. Unpublished position paper. Washington, D.C.: Association of American Medical Colleges.

Weinholtz, D. (1981) *A study of instructional leadership during medical attending rounds.* Unpublished doctoral dissertation, Chapel Hill, N.C.: University of North Carolina.

Weinholtz, D. (1983a). Directing medical student clinical case presentations. *Medical Education,* 17:364–368.

Weinholtz, D. (1983b). Student as attending physician: An instructional innovation. *Journal of Medical Education,* 58(7):590.

Weinholtz, D., and Friedman, C. P. (1985) Conducting qualitative studies using theory and previous research. *Evaluation and the Health Professions,* 8(2):149–176.

Weinholtz, D., and Ostmoe, P. M. (1987) Selecting clinical teaching strategies. In H. Van Hoozer, B. Bratton, P. M. Ostmoe, D. Weinholtz, M. Craft, M. Albanese, and C. Gjerde (eds.): *The teaching process: Theory and practice in nursing.* Norwalk, Conn.: Appleton-Century-Crofts, 173–210.

Weinholtz, D., Friedman, C. P., and Watson, E. (1985) A developmental model for teaching in experiential learning settings. *Professions Education Researcher Notes,* 6(4):3–6.

Weinholtz, D., Albanese, M., Zeitler, R., Everett, G., and Shymansky, J. (1986a) Effective attending physician teaching: The correlation of observed instructional activities and learner ratings of teaching effectiveness. In *Proceedings of the Twenty-Fifth Annual Research in Medical Education Conference.* Washington, D.C.: Association of American Medical Colleges, 273–278.

Weinholtz, D., Freeman, R., and Waickman, A. (1986b) Factors influencing teaching during attending rounds. *Professions Education Researcher Notes,* 7:3–4.

Weinholtz, D., Albanese, M., Zeitler, R., and Everett, G. (1989) Effects of individualized observation with feedback on attending physician teaching. *Teaching and Learning in Medicine,* 1:128–134.

Wilkerson, L., Lesky, L., and Medio, F. J. (1986) The resident as teacher during work rounds. *Journal of Medical Education,* 61:823–829.

Wittrock, M. C. (1986) Students' thought processes. In *Handbook of Research on Teaching.* New York: Macmillan.

Wray, N. P., Friedland, J. A., Ashton, C. M., Scheurich, M. D., and

Zollo, A. J. (1986) Characteristics of house staff work rounds on two academic general medicine services. *Journal of Medical Education,* 61:893–900.

Wylie, N. A. (1988) *The role of the nurse in clinical medical education.* Springfield: Southern Illinois University Press.

INDEX

DONN WEINHOLTZ received his Ph.D. in adult and higher education at the University of North Carolina-Chapel Hill. He is currently the Dean of the College of Education, Nursing, and the Health Professions at the University of Hartford. He has served on the faculties at three medical schools and has been the principal investigator in several studies of teaching in clinical medical education. He edits *Professions Education Researcher Quarterly* for the Education in the Professions Division of the American Educational Research Association.

JANINE C. EDWARDS received her Ph.D. in instructional design from Florida State University's College of Education. She is currently the Director of Research in Medical Education and an associate professor in the Department of Surgery at St. Louis University School of Medicine. She is the author and editor of a number of publications about teaching and learning in clinical settings. Her research interests include graduate medical education, faculty development, and student evaluation in clinical settings.

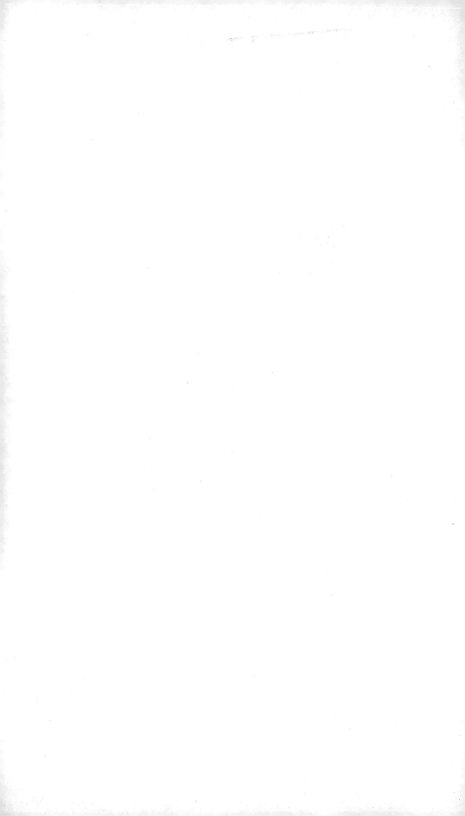